'It's a love story, actually. How people come together in love when it matters, when you hit your rock bottom. It's a love letter to Emma's kids, her family, her friends and her partner, but also to herself. There wasn't one chapter that left me dry-eyed – it's a full-on rollercoaster of a read, and full of Emma's kind soulfulness.'

Grace Timothy, AKA Mum Face Grace, Author

'Meeting Emma and her lovely family really was a moment I won't forget. Such a kind, caring and extremely deserving person. When filming *60 Minute Makeover* we meet many wonderful people and the joy of seeing them receive something that literally can be a turning point in their life is what makes it all worthwhile. She has come through a lot. But now, she has not only proven to be a true fighter, survivor and inspiration, but she's done it with a smile. We may only have met for 60 minutes (give or take 7-10 hours) but she is someone I'll remember for a lifetime.'

Peter Andre

All that followed

Emma Campbell

All that followed

Emma Campbell

A story of cancer, kids
and the fear of leaving too soon

Mirror Books

Published by Mirror Books,
an imprint of Reach plc,
1 Canada Square, London E14 5AP, England

www.mirrorbooks.com
twitter.com/themirrorbooks

Mirror Books 2018

ISBN 978-1-907324-89-5

First paperback edition

Typeset by Danny Lyle
DanJLyle@gmail.com

Printed and bound in Great Britain by
CPI Group (UK) Ltd, Croydon, CR0 4YY

Names and personal details have been changed

Cover images: Richard Payne, iStockphoto

To my four beautiful, crazy,
wild, brilliant angels,
Jake, Ella, Louis and Theo.
I love you more than you could ever know.

And to my darling Dave, my seahorse.
For all the reasons. And all the goodness.

And to all the readers who worry too much.
Who tend to live as though the end is always nigh.
I hope you gain a tiny bit of comfort from
knowing that it's not just you.

contents

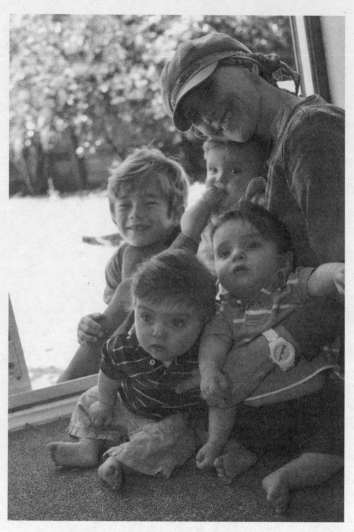

Me and My Four, June 2010.
The cuddles kept me going.

foreword

This book by Emma describes a most remarkable story of fortitude, bravery and courage under the most challenging and extraordinary circumstances.

I first met Emma on the morning of 3rd June 2010. I must have seen tens of thousands of patients presenting with breast cancer, but this was by far the most extraordinary case because of her family circumstances.

She presented to us with a lump. We diagnosed a breast cancer, which needed extensive and complex treatment including multiple drug chemotherapy, radiotherapy and surgery in order to save her life.

The challenging circumstances were that she had four children, triplets born prematurely 5 months previously by Caesarian section and their older brother aged 7. She had breast fed the babies for 3 months but then found the lump in her breast and another under her arm.

Sadly, the partnership with the father of her children broke down and she was then a single parent. She lived in a small flat on the fourth floor with no lift.

Her maternal instincts to live and care for her children were immense.

Would she have the mental courage and physical ability to succeed against these potentially overwhelming challenges?

How could Emma possibly get through all of her treatment and still keep her family together?

It would require a level of determination and a will to prevail, that I could not imagine was possible.

This is her story and her children's story.

Professor Trevor Powles CBE PhD FRCP,
Medical Director, Cancer Centre London (Parkside)

I always knew that one day
I would take this road but
Yesterday
I did not know today
Would be the day.
Nagarjuna

prologue
chelsea and westminster hospital

Notebook Entry, 7 December 2009 (the night before the babies were born)

My life is in freefall.

The stress feels relentless. So much upset clouding the incredible fact that tomorrow morning I'm going to give birth to three babies.

Not sure how I have created/manifested this much chaos and conflict. I dream of life on the other side, of peace in my heart, no more fear.

It feels as though it's over with Marc but the step hasn't been taken. We have broken down completely and my whole being is saying 'no' to us now. How can either of us carry on living like this? Misery, anger, and resentment filling every moment of every day.

Please, please, Marc, realise it too. Let the end be decent.

I must make it my mission to get happy.

For Jake to know Mummy's laugh and to hear it often.

For lightness, silliness, fun.

I want to be free, emotionally free to be the best mum and best me I can possibly be, to shake off all the other rubbish.

To cut the cord with Marc, to say goodbye to that phase of our life together. All the drama, all the conflict.

Is it all my fault?

Is it?

I've found it incredibly hard to shake that thought over the years. On some level, not too far below the surface, I feel responsible for all of it. For the mess that life became. If only I hadn't wanted another baby. If only I'd been able to accept that Jake would be my one and only. If only I hadn't had IVF. If only I hadn't had IVF then maybe the lump wouldn't have turned into cancer and I wouldn't have to live with the constant fear of leaving my babies too soon.

But all of those 'if onlys' would mean that the three most beautiful creatures in the world wouldn't be here. I love you, Jake. I love you, Ella, Louis and Theo. It really was all a bit of a mess for while back there.

I think I've paid the price.

Time to move forward.

chapter one
d-day

Mel's house, Yorkshire, October 2008

'Can you feel that?'

I held Mel's fingers and pushed them into the soft flesh of my right breast, wondering if she could feel the small, hard lump that was most definitely present.

'Hmm, I think so,' she replied, probably not sure what the right answer was. She was cradling her week-old baby in her other arm. I'd taken the train up from London, just for the day, to meet my unofficial goddaughter and to give my best friend a congratulatory hug.

'Would you say it feels like a frozen pea?' Mel asked. She'd had a scare several years before and the doctor had told her that it was the 'hard, like a frozen pea' lumps that we should be concerned about. I wasn't really sure if the lump that I was now so familiar with reminded me of a vegetable. All I knew was that I'd had it for a long time and it niggled me. In hindsight it was wishful thinking, but I just didn't think it could be anything that serious. I was only in my mid-thirties. Far too young for breast cancer, and the GP I'd seen a few months before dismissed it as nothing: 99 per cent sure it's a cyst, she'd said. That was good enough for me. Most of the time.

So once again I pushed the thought of the lump to the back of my mind, cooed over gorgeous baby Jasmine and then at the end of a lovely day, took the train back home.

June 2010. I'll never forget the weather on the day we drove to get the results. It was almost comically dismal. I could imagine an amateur screenwriter drafting the opening scene of a movie with illegible notes scrawled across the script: *torrential rain, dense black cloud. Weather must reflect mood on this dark day.* From what I remember from school it's called pathetic fallacy.

The windscreen wipers worked frantically to reveal the slow traffic ahead but no matter which direction I looked in everything just seemed completely grey. Fifty depressing, varying shades of grey. We drove – Dad, my sister Fiona and me – mostly in silence. Actually, that's a downright lie: I was silent; Dad copes with all situations by talking. He switches between topics with breathtaking ease and somehow we all keep up. I was off the hook that afternoon – nothing expected of me other than my physical presence. I leant back in the passenger seat, eyes closed or else staring at the miserable, strained and, yes, grey faces of weary Londoners, wondering what parallel universe I'd found myself in.

As we stopped and started past the nameless roads and parades of shops I thought about what another mum of six-month-old triplets might be doing with a few precious hours to herself on a rainy Tuesday afternoon. Coffee and cake with an old friend, maybe? Catching up on some much-needed sleep? Or maybe my imaginary multiple mum was at home sorting through a pile of babygros or preparing batches of puréed fruit and vegetables. Maybe her beautiful babies were all snugly strapped into their supersize buggy and being pushed around the park by a caring relative or friend. Just to give mummy a break. Or maybe she was simply sitting down and staring into space. In silence. When you're a mum with several tiny babies and suddenly have some 'you' time, sitting silently and staring into space should not be dismissed as an unprofitable use of that time. As far as I'm concerned it's right up there with being given a foot rub while binge-watching back-to-back episodes of the latest Netflix box set. Anyway, whatever my mythical mummy may or may not have been doing on this particular Tuesday afternoon I could pretty much bet that she wasn't about to be told she had cancer.

In the months that followed Black Tuesday (as it came to be known), it was the mundane that I longed for. Grieved for. Let me be that harassed mother with three screaming babies and an agitated seven-year-old who's picked the wrong queue in Sainsbury's. Let me please have the privilege of going for a routine smear test followed by a trip to the bank and then the garage because the car's failed its MOT. Please, let life be ordinary.

So, there was something comforting about the chatter of my sister and father as we neared St Helier Hospital. The familiarity of their voices, the way they sparked off each other, their sharp minds and quick wit always leaving me trailing behind, the passionate declarations that we'd all get through this 'fucking nightmare', and one of Dad's favourite lines: 'You won't know yourself a year from now, my darling! You'll look back on all this and –'

And what? I wondered. I felt so exhausted by life already – could I really find the extra strength required to enter into a lengthy battle with cancer?

We turned off the main road and into the small but full hospital car park, squeezing Dad's battered old Peugeot 305 in between a clapped-out silver Volvo Estate and a shiny four-by-four that had one of those annoying *Baby on Board* signs stuck in the back. Dad turned off the engine and we just sat there for a moment. Silent. The babies' faces were everywhere I looked. The boys' giant eyes. Louis's anxious, permanently troubled expression. Ella's nose, so soft, small and squishy that it looked like it had melted in the sun. Theo's ridiculously easy smile. And Jake – my big boy, Jake. Not so big, actually, at barely seven years old, but bigger than his triplet siblings and therefore somehow expected to behave like a young adult or a father figure, or… something. *Big brother Jake. Look after your mother, Jake. Be a good boy for Mummy, Jake.* Already far more demanded of him than was fair. This day would push him even further away from the carefree childhood he used to know, further than I could bear to think about.

We were due to see the consultant at 5 p.m. and I'd been told I was his last appointment of the day. This apparently trivial piece of information somehow seemed significant to me – my *look for the negative in everything* antennae in fine working order. Being given the last slot of the day quite clearly only meant one thing. Bad news.

We were there so early it was ridiculous. Talk about prolonging the agony. I always get everywhere early. Even being precisely on time makes me anxious and edgy. Dad and Fiona do not share this trait and probably, on this particular occasion, I would have been wise to follow their lead and not insist that we allow ninety minutes to make a forty-minute journey. But the babies and Jake were all in good hands and hey, we multiple mums need to take time out when and where we can.

St Helier Hospital is a stone's throw away from a local hospice and I think the three of us felt like death had tapped us on the shoulder when we eventually got out of the car and looked around for the entrance. *You look a bit lost!* I imagined Death saying, wide-grinned like Jim Carrey in *The Mask. Not to worry, I'll show you the way. It's straight ahead through those double doors of doom, along the corridor that's adorned with crucifixes and you'll find hell's waiting room is just on your left. We've saved you a seat; I'll be along right behind you.*

As we walked down the long corridor it struck me that silence really could be deafening. It's the noise of isolation, the voices in your head. Was this really a hospital? Where were the patients? The atmosphere seemed so still, so civilised with its pale-carpeted floors, freshly painted walls and plug-in air fresheners jutting out of every other socket. I visibly shuddered as the three of us took our seats at the far end of the waiting area. Dad and I sat next to each other and it felt completely natural to reach for his hand just as I've always done. I love Dad's hands. Shaped beautifully by decades of hard work and a lifetime of artistic brilliance. The simple gold ring he's always worn on the little finger of his left hand, his warm, strong grip, squeezing my fingers tightly. I might as well have been six years old again. With Dad here, surely everything would be alright? There was almost nothing in my life so far that he hadn't been able to fix, nothing he hadn't been able to make better. The only safe harbour I'd ever known, my dad.

We caught each other's eyes and he gave me a big smile and squeezed my cold fingers once again. I was shivering as the anxiety took hold. *Don't you worry, my darling, it's all going to be fine,* cheering me on as always. But there was no denying it; today he looked shattered. Fiona sat to our left, fidgety and restless. My big sis, my best sis, my only sis. Seven years between us, and so different to each other, but as close as two sisters can be. My confidante, my teaser and tormenter. They were the only two I needed that day. They were going to make sure everything was OK. Their fierce, protective love wrapped itself around me as we sat and stared ahead and then at each other. What on earth were we doing here? What the hell was going on? The nervous laughter set in.

I was reminded of my grandad's funeral. I was seventeen, Fiona twenty-four. In a small church in a tiny village called Back, on the Isle of Lewis in the Outer Hebrides. We sat in the row behind my grandmother and the many members of Grandad's family – none of whom Grandma had much time for. Apart from Auntie Annie, that was. 'Annie's all right,' she would say in her broad Geordie accent, puffing away in a cloud of Super Kings.

That was another day when the weather mirrored events. The wind was fierce and the rain relentless. The sermon was long, dramatic and really quite frightening, real fire and brimstone stuff. We'd spent a heartbreaking week by Grandad's side, sent up by Dad to be there during his final days. Grandma was angry and disconnected so we were the ones who sat by the deathbed as he drifted in and out of fitful sleep. We were the ones who put those funny little pink foam mouth swabs soaked in water into his parched, sore mouth and softly whispered to him for seven days and nights. Grandma was cross that we wouldn't leave his side.

'You're here to help me!' she stormed angrily, crashing pots and pans around in the kitchen. No. We were there to soothe the final days of a dying man. A man we'd never really got to know but who we loved anyway.

It had been such a strange week, unlike anything we'd ever experienced. Despite my grandfather's rejection of the Free Church of Scotland, every passing visitor or district nurse would mumble lines from the Bible and talk of forgiveness and sin and of course there was a wake after he died. Locals from the village, fishermen with weatherbeaten faces stood and sang strange Gaelic songs of mourning in the living room and then sat down with a cup of tea and a chocolate wafer and talked about fish, peat and, of course, the weather. Fiona and I were the *Sassanachs*. Two English girls who didn't really belong. By this point Fiona had been a Buddhist for six years and the closest I got to any kind of formal religion was devouring every self-help book I could lay my hands on.

By the time the congregation had all taken their seats in the church for the service and the minister began his sermon it was just too much for us and we exploded into helpless, mortifying laughter. Tears streamed down our faces as we sat in our pews, breathlessly hysterical – silent, painful laugher that teetered between mirth and misery.

So, as the three of us sat in the waiting room that day I wasn't remotely offended that Fiona was enjoying what may well have been the best laugh she'd had in years. Or that Dad's shoulders were shuddering so much that two tiny tears had appeared at the corner of each eye. At least I think they were tears of laughter. It was all too much. Here I was, dragging everyone I loved through this hell, so I was strangely comforted by the knowledge that laughter – nervous, inappropriate or whatever – was still a possibility. The horrendous wait we'd had to endure over the last few days had been agony for us all. The anxiety had to be released somehow; it's just that, personally, I couldn't imagine myself ever laughing again.

After what seemed like an eternity, the consultant appeared. I'd met him for the first time four days earlier after an appointment with the local GP had quickly escalated into a shit-there's-clearly-something-wrong-here type of situation. Which I'd known anyway, deep down. I just hadn't been able to face dealing with it because of everything else. Unable to stand the thought of waiting two weeks for a referral, I'd managed to get an emergency appointment privately, thanks to the medical cover I had through work. And so, on the Friday afternoon just before the May bank holiday weekend, I found myself having blood tests, a biopsy and a very serious talk with a man who was going to feature heavily in my life over the coming months: Mr Sharma.

He ushered us into his office and we all took a seat, me in the middle between Dad and Fiona again. I waited for the bomb to drop and drop it most certainly did. No polite chit-chat: Mr Sharma got straight to the point. 'It is a cancer we're dealing with,' he said calmly and then paused to give us a moment.

Despite this being the news we'd spent the last few days preparing ourselves to hear we still sat stunned, staring at him with absolutely no idea of what to say. *A cancer.* That sounded so strange to me. What did he mean by 'a' cancer? Wasn't cancer just cancer? I knew nothing then. Knew nothing of the world I was being shoved into whether I liked it or not.

'There's a good chance we can cure it,' he continued pragmatically. 'But it's going to be a long road ahead.'

Good chance? I thought. *Good chance?!* The words spun around in my head and once again, those dancing images of my three babies and Jake. I needed a whole lot more than a good chance. I needed certainty.

Mr Sharma continued to speak. 'The tumour is rather large so the likely plan is that we'll start you off with eight cycles of chemotherapy to shrink it. This will give us a better chance of success when we perform the mastectomy.

'We'll perform a reconstruction at the same time and then, after a period of recovery, you'll follow on with several weeks of daily radiotherapy which will blast away any stray cancer cells that might have been left behind. You may need further chemotherapy after that, we'll have to see.'

Visions of multi-coloured headscarves filled my head, Gypsy Rose Lee lookalikes wearing big hooped earrings. This was really happening. I was about to become someone completely different. A new Emma I had no desire to meet.

The rest of the conversation was a blur. Fiona asked questions and took notes on my behalf. Apparently 'my' cancer (the cancer I did not want to own) was HER2-positive, but would respond to a drug called Herceptin and chemotherapy. The cancer was also hormone receptor positive and should respond to the drug Tamoxifen.

This information meant absolutely nothing to me. Mr Sharma could have been talking in Latin for all the sense it made. More blood tests and scans were arranged, after which we would apparently know *exactly* what we were dealing with. I was so naive back then that I didn't realise that meant we would know whether or not the cancer had spread.

'I'm going to arrange for you to meet with Professor Trevor Powles later on this week. He'll be your oncologist.'

I didn't even know what an oncologist was.

'He's one of the best in the business,' Mr Sharma said with a certain amount of pride, as the three of us just stared blankly back at him. He went on tell us that Trevor and his identical twin brother Ray, also an oncologist, had been on *This Is Your Life* several years earlier, applauded for their pioneering work. My addled brain was then immediately flooded with childhood memories of Wednesday night, pre-*Coronation Street* episodes of what was a truly iconic TV show – famously hosted by Eamonn Andrews and his Big Red

Book. I imagined Eamonn – who seemed like a lovely, gentle giant of a man – putting his hand on my shoulder and saying in his soft Irish brogue, *'Tonight, Emma, this is your life.'* 'Er, thanks, Eamonn,' I'd reply, no doubt turning a bit pink and flustered at all the attention, *'but it hasn't quite turned out as planned…'*

Mr Sharma tried to end our meeting on a positive note.

'Look, I could be telling you to go on a round-the-world cruise,' he said, smiling gently. 'And I'm not saying that.' I now had visions of P&O Cruises, all-you-could-eat buffets and *Take That* tribute acts floating through my brain. It seemed like my mind wanted to focus on every irrelevant aside rather than the main topic for discussion. We smiled politely, stood up, shook hands, and agreed to meet again in two days' time to discuss the latest test results and plan the first part of my treatment.

On the way home, Dad was on a strange kind of high, salvaging what he could from the wreckage. He and Fiona talked even more quickly and randomly, both near euphoric that there seemed to be some hope, clearly relieved that all was not lost and that I could, if I wanted, fight this thing.

Once again, I just let them talk. I had reverted to child mode and had nothing to say. All I could think about were the faces of my little angels at home. My three little darlings, too tiny, thank God, to have a clue what was going on. But what about my Jakey? My gorgeous nature boy - never happier than when he's catching the frogs and toads in Grandad's garden pond with his bare hands or examining the insects that hide beneath the broken paving slabs on the path. How could I look him in the eye? What would I say, how could I possibly explain what lay ahead? His world had already been turned upside down in the last few months and he'd been strong and adapted so well. How was he going to cope with Mummy being ill on top of it all?

chapter two
memories and two double-yolkers

I remember lying on the grass on a hot June afternoon. Thirty-one years old. Jeans hanging loose, appetite gone, living on red wine and bowls of chips in cozy French bistros. Days blurring into one. We were one of those sickeningly happy couples – unselfconscious and engrossed in each other. Newly in love.

'What were you doing when you were twenty? Twenty-five? Twenty-six?'

Question after question you'd ask during those early days and weeks, wanting to know the fragments of my life, wanting to climb into my past and claim it as your own. I remember listening to David Bowie and trying to disguise a red raw chin, bleeding and sore from days spent kissing.

You thought the years before we met had been wasted; I knew the Plain Jane me from before would never have caught the eye of a handsome Parisian whose looks led the way.

I remember a vivid blue line on a stick there was no need to buy. Too soon, surely this was all too soon.

I remember moments. Spinning through my head, over and over. What was the real us? The good or the bad? Moments of perfection and moments of hell.

I remember Jake's first night. Our angel was here. We were both instantly in love. The world felt good and so did we.

I remember spooning and watching Jonathan Ross and belly button fluff and lost jobs and silent meal times. I remember extremes, a see-saw of good and bad, a constant analysis – lost hours spent weighing up the right against the wrong. Of a relationship feeding on itself.

I remember lying in bed alone as the sun came up.

I remember not recognizing the screaming banshee I'd become, leaping around in front of your swaying form, demanding answers and apologies.

I remember the night we agreed to make three become four. Little did we know what lay in wait. And then I remember a longing so deep and so physical that it consumed me and damaged us. Just one more baby. I could think of nothing else. Please, just one more baby. Three devastating losses over as many years that only made me more crazy and obsessed. If I could just have another baby then I could cope with anything. I mean it – anything. I used to look up and stare defiantly at the sky. I used to challenge the universe, not realising it was listening.

'Bring it on,' I seemed to be saying to God, the moon, the stars and you.

I remember tangled limbs on a flickering screen, grainy black and white ghosts, hearing that three had become six. Triplets. The world stopped, our fragile universe tilted. I caught your eye: pure shock, and pure panic.

Our boy Jake punched the air and cried, 'Yes!' and the man in the long white coat wiped the gel from my tight, swollen belly and looked grave.

I remember pure fear. I remember knowing we would crumble.

Three little treasures waiting in the wings. Perfect, glowing little bundles, each bringing love and each carrying a hand grenade.

Our final chapter had begun.

It was a bright, sunny Sunday morning in April 2009. On that particular morning, we were okay. Marc was making breakfast, Steve Wright was playing his Sunday love songs and there was a feeling of harmony between us that I never took for granted. Jake was five and bouncing around in our large, bright kitchen. The kitchen that used to be a neglected balcony on the side of the top-floor, one-bedroom flat I'd called home for so many years. The sparkling new kitchen that had meant we could finally give our boy his own room and us some much-needed space. The kitchen that made us seem like real grown-ups as we made coffee and slathered salty butter onto fresh, warm bread. I laid the table as Jake chattered and darted around us, our bundle of goodness, always filling in the gaps, his very existence making us seem more solid than we were.

Marc liked to cook. He cooked with tremendous confidence and concentration. His handsome face would become serious and it was one of the rare times when there wasn't a Marlboro Light dangling from the corner of his mouth. He didn't seem to appreciate being interrupted as he focused on whichever dish he was creating, and this didn't fit in with my fantasy of idle chit-chat and closeness. I always craved conversation when we were together. 'Talk to me,' I'd say as the three of us sat in silence at breakfast or lunch or dinner. I dreamt of chatter and noise and the chaos of a large family with mum and dad at the helm, united and strong. Talking, talking all the time, their deep-rooted love regularly watered with shared jokes, banter and intimate asides.

'I eat, Emma,' Marc would say, head down and brow furrowed. And I would turn to Jake and engage in more talk of *Fireman Sam* and horses and dinosaurs or whatever his current obsessions were. It wasn't Marc's fault, of course. No need to talk just for the sake of it. It was just what I yearned for.

This was a good morning. I'd already been up with Jake for hours, drinking endless cups of tea while he watched back-to-back episodes of *Octonauts*. Marc eventually emerged with bedhead hair and a crinkled smile and headed straight to the coffee machine for an espresso to go with his first cigarette of the day. He was between jobs but, as always, I did my best to put the stress that caused to one side and tried my damnedest not to voice the nagging concerns that were niggling away, or ask any of the tense, provocative little questions I had about how our future, because I just wanted us to be okay.

I made sure we were okay a lot of the time because I wanted another baby so much. Everybody around us knew it. They must have whispered and mumbled sympathetically as the months and years passed and I went a little bit mad.

Secondary infertility sent me off the rails. It really did. For nearly four long years it dominated every waking thought I had, affected every choice I made and changed the way I lived. It changed me. It was all consuming and so, by default, it consumed others too, dominating my closest relationships – and for that I feel a sense of shame. Or if shame is too strong a word, embarrassment at least. I was a woman obsessed. *Just one more baby*. To me, it was simple. My life, our life, would be complete with One. More. Baby.

My kids. The kids. The kids are driving me mad. Got to pick the kids up from swimming. Kids! Will you PLEASE stop fighting!

I wanted what I imagined to be the everyday chaos of life with two children. I wanted it for Jake. At least that's what I told myself and anybody else who'd listen.

"Jake needs a brother or a sister," I'd say, as yet another conversation was led by my longing. I realise now that Jake was fine. He was more than fine. He was a happy, sunshine-filled little boy with golden curls and the gentlest temperament I'd ever known. The closest Jake ever got to a tantrum was a bit of mild whining when I said no to another custard cream. I look back now and know that I really was in the grip of a kind of madness. A madness that, now I'm out the other side, I struggle to understand. But maybe that's because I got my second baby. And my third baby. And my fourth. I didn't mean to be greedy. I didn't ever mean for Ella, Louis and Theo to think that their arrival precipitated an earthquake in our world.

I learned to appreciate the good moments between Marc and me. Those are what kept me going. There was an essential decency between us; there was a love of sorts. A love I thought at the time was solid and real but was actually fragile, volatile and, at its core, unseaworthy.

So cooking a fry-up on a sunny spring morning a few weeks before we were due to start IVF treatment, and feeling upbeat and hopeful that something good was about to happen in our lives, were nice feelings to have.

'You want scrambled eggs, my love?' asked Marc from his position at the stove, not looking up as he reached for the pan and threw a tea towel over his shoulder.

'Fried, please,' I replied, picking Jake up and holding him close. He was too big now to be carried but I could never resist and he never complained. I walked over to where Marc was cooking, put my arm around his waist and leant in to him, feeling content. He cracked the first egg into the pan and we all did a little gasp, just like when you're stuck in a traffic jam and it's been raining all day and suddenly you look up and see a rainbow. Has anyone, ever, in the history of rainbows, not gasped at a rainbow?

'Wow! Look at that!' I cried. 'Look, Jakey, that's a double yolker!'

'How does that happen, Mummy?'

'Er, let's Google it, sweetheart.' I replied, using the default response I found myself relying on more with each passing day.

'Do it again, Papa!'

We laughed, knowing there was no way it would happen twice in a row. But an air of anticipation began to form, nevertheless. Marc reached for a second egg and the three of us leaned over the pan again, waiting. It was a bit like that moment in *Charlie and the Chocolate Factory* when there's only one Golden Ticket left. Charlie and Grandpa Joe sit together on the rickety old bed, skinny, starving and holding their breath as Charlie carefully peels back the shiny wrapper, not knowing this is the moment when their lives change forever.

And there they were. Two more perfect golden circles, nestled next to each other like it was the most natural thing in the world. Like they belonged together. It felt like a miracle to me. Of course, at the time, I didn't know that double yolks are caused by an over-stimulated ovary in the hen. I didn't know much about ovaries at all, other than that mine weren't working very well.

'Well,' I declared triumphantly, putting Jake down and running my fingers through his thick darkening blonde hair before he ducked away and ran off. 'That's it then, you two. There's no doubt about it. We're definitely having quads.'

Jake took me at my word and whooped around the kitchen, chanting the future names of all the babies he'd also decided we were definitely going to have. I smiled a little too brightly at Marc and tried to keep the moment light.

'What if we have twins, Emma?' he would ask on a regular basis, gesturing upstairs to our two tiny bedrooms and inhaling sharply on another cigarette. 'Where will we put two babies?'

'Twins?!' I would reply, dismissing him out of hand. 'Don't be ridiculous,' I'd say, sighing at a question I thought barely warranted an answer. 'You know what the odds of IVF are. It'll be an absolute miracle if we have one baby, let alone two.'

We all sat down and enjoyed a delicious breakfast, although I did feel a bit strange about eating our magic eggs. Again, Marc ate in silence. Jake chatted nonstop about his favourite animals and I added his questions to my never-ending mental list of stuff to look up online later on. It was a Sunday morning I've never forgotten. Little did we know then that my innocent but soon to be over-stimulated ovaries were about to get the shock of their lives.

chapter three
how we began

When I found out I was pregnant with Jake I was terrified and briefly devastated. Ironic, eh? Marc and I had only been together for five months; he'd officially moved in after a few short weeks and we were having a ball. Weekends in bed, romantic strolls in the park, endless bottles of red wine, an introduction to French music and a new appreciation of rich, buttery, creamy *fromage*-filled culinary delights that should have been expanding my waistline by the day but weren't because... well, use your imagination.

I was in love and so was he and because of that I didn't think too much about the incompatibilities that might cause problems between us at some point. I was completely swept away by his gorgeous crinkly-eyed smile, his gentle hands, his laugh and the declarations of love, true love that seemed so sincere.

We talked very early on, first date early on in actual fact, about both wanting babies. Obviously not with each other at that point (hey, I was playing it cool) but I remember him asking me if I wanted children one day and when I replied with a definite yes he smiled that smile, said *me too* and just left it there. He held my gaze for so long that I thought I was going to pass out and the cheese burger and chunky chips I'd been toying with were pushed away. Lovesick. Smitten. From the word go.

Marc and I had first met when he was working in my favourite little writing spot in Clapham. A French bistro called *Gastro*, just opposite the Picture House cinema on Venn Street. Once or twice a week I'd sit in a corner table, notebook out, hot coffee to my right, and simply scribble away. For hours. No tablets, MacBooks, no Instagram story distractions. It was a prolific time; I must have filled a dozen A5 notebooks in as many months. With what, I'm not quite sure – but hey, at least I was doing what I loved most.

It was April or May 2002 and I'd just turned thirty-one. I guess I was ready. Ready for something. So one afternoon, as the sun went down and the handsome waiter who'd served me a café au lait leant over and lit the tea light on my table, I glanced up and 'something' happened.

'It's more romantic,' he said with the most pronounced French accent I'd ever heard. Smiling, his green eyes held my gaze as the flame softly flickered and he put his lighter back in pocket of his apron.

He must have known that would have an effect. And boy. It certainly did.

For the next few weeks, every time I returned, it was all about the eye contact. Oh, the eye contact. Is there anything more delicious than looking up to find that the person you're infatuated with staring right at you? And he was so handsome! And I was so lacking in confidence! And so, so ready to be swept off my feet by an *extremely* charming Parisian called Marc.

We finally got chatting one Sunday afternoon. I'd dragged my friend Sophie along to keep me company and the two of us sat eking out a bowl of chips and a couple of hot chocolates each (which then turned to glasses of house red) for what seemed like hours. Then, eventually and much to my intense delight, Marc took a break and sat about a foot away from our table at the bar, nursing a tall, bright green beverage. I tried extremely hard to keep focused on whatever conversation it was Sophie and I were having but she knew the score. She was *well* aware that I had an agenda that afternoon, that I needed my buddy with me while I tried ascertain if I really had made an impression on this handsome waiter or if his subtle flirting was just his 'way' with the female clientele. Soph played her part to absolute perfection.

'Excuse me, what's that drink called?' She said, nodding to the emerald green drink in his hands.

And that was that.

Bang. Conversation started. What a genius. Within minutes, Marc had joined us at our table and there he stayed until his next shift started an hour or so later. Once his break was over and he was back to work, Sophie and I ended up staying on for something to eat. We drank more wine and I enjoyed even more intense eye contact with Marc. By about nine o'clock Sophie had more than done her bit and decided to call it a night.

'Thank you! Thank you soooo much!' I whispered in her ear as we hugged our goodbyes.

'Call me tomorrow,' she winked back while putting on her coat. 'And have fun.'

It was nearly midnight by the time Marc turned the 'open' sign to 'closed' on the door and midnight by the time he and I leapt into a cab to the Fridge bar in Brixton where we did our best to talk over the thumping beat of a heavy mix of nineties R'n'B and Garage.

Sitting at the bar we kissed and it was lovely. At one point we started talking about horoscopes and I took it as a sign, a definite sign, that Marc shared his birthday with Mel's brother Miles (who's like the brother I never had.) Then bizarrely, and I swear I'd only been on the wine, we sat comparing our thumbs. We decided that they were absolutely identical. Identical thumbs. We were quite clearly a match made in heaven.

So we started seeing each other and I was very, very happy. Marc left Gastro within a week of us meeting but it didn't worry me too much. I could probably cover things for a while. Our endless meals out, our bottles of wine. Our overspending at the local deli for yet another candlelit feast at the flat. It would all balance out, I was sure. Anyway, Marc had a plan – the restaurant jobs were a stopgap. I had to admire him: he'd only been in London a few months, was finding his way and that was way more than I'd ever done in another country – I hadn't ever lived outside the postcode I was born in.

Meanwhile, I was temping by day and attending writing classes at night. When Marc and I met I'd just written a trial script for the Channel 5 soap *Family Affairs* and as I hadn't yet had it rejected I was in a pretty positive, hopeful place. I felt as though I could legitimately call myself a writer – a feeling that wouldn't last long at all.

I can barely remember the heady early days of our relationship now. They were lovely but far too brief. But I do remember the first time I met his parents, Alain and Nicolette. They visited from Paris and we had a pleasant getting-to-know-each-other weekend of sightseeing, exhibitions and more meals out. Although the conversation didn't exactly flow, given their faltering English and my non-existent French, it definitely felt like a significant step forward in mine and Marc's relationship. Parents met: tick. They seemed nice, from what I could tell.

On the Monday morning, we saw them off at Waterloo Station (back in the day when it was the Eurostar's home). Alain gave me a big hug goodbye and then said something I've never forgotten.

'I hope you love very much this bad boy.'

He then squeezed me one last time before turning away and, really, it almost felt as though he was thanking me.

I couldn't quite put my finger on it, but I had the distinct feeling that Alain and Nicolette were returning to their little corner of Paris feeling very, very relieved that all was well in the world of their son, Marc, and his new London girl, Emma.

And the rest, as they say, is history. And what a complicated history it is.

chapter four
first time round

When Marc and I first became an item, my naivety knew no bounds. After years of stumbling around in the relationship desert, being sensible was not at the forefront of my hungry and ever so slightly dirty mind. The contraceptive pill was not an option based on my one attempt at taking it a few years earlier – a ten-pound weight gain within as many days and more suicidal thoughts than I knew what to do with made it an absolute no-no a second time round. Condoms were given short shrift very early on and so we found ourselves taking the ridiculous route of simply 'being careful'.

'What are you using, condoms or the pill?' close girl friends would ask over wine and a catch-up.

'Oh,' I'd reply, shrugging nonchalantly. 'We're just being careful.'

What a joke that was. When it comes to making babies there ain't no such thing and so really it was only a matter of time before I found myself stopping at the Waterloo Station branch of Boots on the way home from work and purchasing a pregnancy test. I'd barely got back to the flat and taken my coat off before I locked myself in the bathroom and ripped the damn thing open. Marc waited for me in the kitchen, chewing his nails and just about managing not to break our 'no smoking inside the flat' rule.

Whoosh. The blue line appeared instantly. It couldn't have been more blue. Pregnant. One hundred per cent pregnant. Without. Even. Trying.

We were both shell-shocked, despite having no right to be. Marc held me as I cried in his arms that night. Not yet, not yet. It was simply too soon. I wasn't ready to give up 'us' – being a young couple newly in love, the honeymoon period, the spontaneity. Forget our low incomes, debt and floundering, non-existent careers. Forget the fact that we'd only been together a short time – and was I really absolutely sure that we were a good match?

None of the sensible stuff crossed my mind. I loved Marc and we could get round all the practicalities. It was just too soon. I'd only just finally cast aside my solitary status and I was gutted, *gutted* that our 'love's young dream' phase was going to be over, or at the very least so dramatically altered, so prematurely.

Those fearful feelings were fleeting. Within days I had completely come round to the idea, we both had, and along with intense nausea and fatigue, euphoria set in. A baby. Our baby. Our little bilingual bundle. We were going to be a family! Maybe we'd go and live close to his parents and sister in Paris for a while. Marc would find work that made him happy and I, while nurturing our *petit ange*, would write a book, or script, or children's story, anything. I'd write, I'd be a writer and our world would be a good one.

The pregnancy wasn't easy. At fifteen weeks I was rushed to hospital with what seemed to be a miscarriage. There was no pain but a horrific amount of blood. I was admitted overnight and booked for an emergency scan the following morning. 'Suspected miscarriage' was written on my admission notes and the hospital chaplain came to visit us as I rested in bed.

When I was finally wheeled down to the ultrasound unit and placed on the bed, jellied up and holding tightly onto Marc's hand, I couldn't look.

'Turn the screen away,' I pleaded, tears streaming down my face. 'I don't want to see.' Just three weeks earlier we'd celebrated a healthy twelve-week scan – the big pregnancy milestone. It was real, it was happening and I was already in love. And now it was over. Our baby had gone.

There was a tense silence for a few moments. Marc squeezed my hand tightly and stroked my hair. The radiographer swirled the strobe on my gently swollen belly and we waited to hear the heartbreaking words that would confirm our loss.

'And there's the baby's heartbeat. Nice and strong.'

We looked at the screen and there was our baby as alive as alive could be. Disco dancing, jiving like a junior John Travolta. There was Jake, our apple-sized boy.

The remainder of the pregnancy was physically smooth and steady but my anxiety levels were not. I was terrified of having another bleed and found it virtually impossible to relax and enjoy the experience. And Marc and I really weren't in a great place. Our relationship, still so new, was already being tested in a way that neither of us had expected.

The good days/bad days/good nights/hellish nights pattern of our relationship was firmly established during the final weeks before Jake was born. Cemented into the DNA of Marc and Emma. We had become 'that' couple and the haphazard, far from healthy way that we functioned together, unfortunately, never really changed.

But, despite our failings, there can be no doubt that we created pure goodness in the form of Jake. Born four weeks early by emergency caesarian section on a warm Wednesday evening, just as London was entering one of its hottest summers on record, Jake had a hold on my heart from the start. It was an instant soul connection. Solid, unbreakable and like nothing I'd ever experienced. As I held him in my arms on that first night, his deep, dark blue, saucer-shaped eyes bored into mine and the love I felt took my breath away. My soul floated down into his gaze and he had me. He still does.

Unfortunately, the time that Marc and I spent in our bubble of new baby bliss was cut short in a totally unexpected and terrifying way.

The first twenty-fours were pretty textbook. I was a bit sore from the c-section, obviously very tired but nothing that you wouldn't expect after giving birth. Visitors and midwives popped in and out, all cooing over our gorgeous boy, the doctors did their morning rounds and glanced quickly at the stitches on my tummy before moving as quickly as was polite onto the lady in the next bed.

By the Thursday night I really wasn't feeling well at all. I was feverish and freezing with what I suppose you could describe as flu-like symptoms. Except my abdomen was also sore. So sore in fact that I wanted to scream if anyone went near it. Having never had a baby before, let alone any kind of major abdominal surgery, I didn't know what was normal so I didn't say too much and no doctors or nurses asked. Maybe this was par for the course? Maybe being in agony after a c-section was just another of the many *real* truths of motherhood that had been kept from me? I tried to block out the pain and focus on Jake and the frustrating task of trying to get his tiny little mouth to latch onto one of my flat, inverted and extremely uncooperative nipples.

It was virtually impossible to get any kind of sleep that night. Aside from the pain I was in, the half a dozen or so newborn babies on the post-natal ward had clearly made some kind of pre-birth pact to cry in shifts. All the midwives on duty were gathered around their workstation and seemed to be having an impromptu party, and the unforgiving fluorescent strips that lit the corridor cast a cold, intrusive light into the ward, making it utterly impossible to drift off.

I was feeling worse by the minute and suddenly it was clear that I urgently needed to be sick. I pressed the alarm by the side of the bed to call one of the midwives but to no avail. When I eventually managed to inch myself off the bed, up onto my feet and stagger out of the ward towards them, it appeared as though they had far more pressing matters to attend to. I can't really blame them – I've certainly never managed to sit near an open tin of Quality Streets and not give it my full focus and concentration to the exclusion of everything else going on around me.

Foraging for the purples and disdainfully casting aside the strawberry and orange fondants, it seemed as though they were far too busy to notice a young woman in an untied and open-backed hospital gown, shuffling over to one of the small sinks opposite their desk. I couldn't hold it in. I couldn't see anything else; there certainly weren't any random buckets lying around. It was the sink or the floor. I chose the sink. Bad idea.

I was spotted by one of the nurses just as she realised she'd accidentally bitten into the yucky coconut one (surely the least popular of all the 'Streets'?) and she was not a happy bunny.

'Do you mind not being sick into the sink, please?' she said crossly.

'Sorry,' I mumbled, suddenly feeling horribly vulnerable and close to tears. We both glanced at the contents of the sink. It was dark, green and unlike anything I'd ever seen come out of my mouth before. I pulled some paper out of the dispenser on the wall and wiped my face before inching my way slowly back to bed. The nausea had subsided but the searing pain in my stomach had not.

The next morning a bright and bubbly lady from the discharge team came round to see me with a clipboard and a form to sign.

'You can go home later today, Emma! If you just sign here we'll process your discharge and you and baby should be out by mid afternoon.'

It was nearly a month before 'baby' and I got to go home. That night I found myself in an operating theatre being given an emergency tracheotomy and being prepared for the first of several life-saving operations.

By the time it was properly diagnosed eleven days later, necrotising fasciitis – a flesh-eating bug that surely must be the subject of its own *Hammer House of Horror* movie – had done its very best to try and gobble me up. Literally. Google it, click on images and you'll see some real sights. YouTube it and you'll probably want to give dinner a miss.

A year or so later, when the physical scars were slowly healing but the mental trauma lingered on, I stumbled upon an episode of *Oprah* in which she interviewed a woman with no limbs. This thirty-something mother of two spoke of her inspirational recovery from 'nec fash' (as we in the know call it) and the audience were shown an awe-inspiring piece of pre-recorded footage that demonstrated how, despite having no arms or legs, she still managed to cook dinner every night for her family and get her kids dressed and ready for school in the mornings.

There really are no words to say to that. I lost the flesh on my stomach, have a fake belly button and a perfect rectangle on my right thigh where skin was grafted on to my stomach, but I still have my limbs.

I have scars on the top of my legs where drains were inserted to try and prevent a build-up of toxic fluid and halt further infection but I can still walk and, God help them, I can still cook for my children using the hands I was born with.

Funny though – after a lifetime spent facing a million imaginary deaths, Jake's birth led to my very first brush with the real thing.

Do you want to know what else is funny? There's nothing like a birth trauma to make you hell-bent on doing the whole pregnancy thing all over again and this time being absolutely determined to get it right.

chapter five
desperate times

Diary Entry, Spring 2009

Dear Jake,

I'm so sorry that I haven't been able to give you a brother or sister yet. I want more than anything to make it happen. I haven't been a very good mum today. I've felt irritable, harsh and locked into my own thoughts and feelings – not giving you the attention you deserve.

This morning you were playing alone in your room. As I paused outside your bedroom door you seemed happy, in your own little world. It sounded like you were having a conversation. You're five years old with a vivid imagination so I know that's nothing out of the ordinary. If you had a sibling, I wouldn't give a second thought to that scene. But you don't, so I worry that you're talking aloud because you're lonely, because you have no real lifelong 'mate' to squabble with, wake up with and share secret thoughts with. It makes my heart ache. I feel like I'm depriving you of something so amazing – something you would take totally for granted if you had it, of course. But because you don't, it seems like there's a gaping hole, a missing piece in the jigsaw of your life.

I'm projecting, of course. All of my 'stuff' onto your gorgeous little head. Something is missing for me and so I presume it is for you too. Is it? Do you feel the lack like I do? We were supposed to start IVF treatment this weekend. A blood test has revealed my body hasn't played ball this month so treatment is delayed. After three and a half years we're finally ready so this hitch in the plans has hit me hard and I don't know what to do with myself today, or with you.

Becca just phoned to confirm our plans for next week – we're taking you all to the theatre which will be fun. I asked her what she was up to today and she said that her, Tony and the boys were spending a lazy day at home together, just pottering about. I put the phone down and wanted to cry. You, Papa and I are a triangle – a tight, loving triangle (most of the time!) – but two sides are aching to open out and welcome in the missing piece. To me, a family is square-shaped, with four sides.

I needed to put some of this down in writing tonight. My chest is tight with unexpressed thoughts, fears and rubbish. I just want another baby. I want to know that I've done it, that I'm standing on the other side of the mountain and that whatever else life throws at us (as it no doubt will), we are done. That our family is complete, with Mummy, Papa, Jake – and our missing piece.

I love you so much, Jakey, and I'm so sorry if all of this baby stuff stops me from being the mother I should be. You are my world, my universe and you deserve the best of me.

Always and forever,
Mummy XXX

You don't just 'try' IVF. You don't just casually 'give it a go'. Fertility treatment comes at the end of a painfully long road. It comes after treacherous disappointment and loss and after the longing for a baby has drained the joy out of life and the life out of your relationship. So, by the time one year of trying to conceive had become two, and two years had become nearly four, and by the time we'd recovered from the three pregnancies that had ended just after they'd begun, we were not solid, really not solid at all.

I was home alone the night before the I was due to have my eggs harvested at the fertility clinic and Marc was expected to produce a sample and hand it to the nearest nurse waving a petri dish. The plan being that one of my carefully cultivated eggs and one of his Tom Daley champion swimmers would meet, merge, live happily ever after and we would have our baby. Simple. After weeks of daily blood tests, scans, a cocktail of hormones and injections with needles so big that I am now the proud owner of my very own phobia, my ovaries had done their best and we were ready.

I say 'we'. I was ready. Terrified but ready. The emotions surrounding the whole 'hot' topic fluctuated all the time between Marc and me. There were many good, hopeful, united phases of a shared vision and a dream fulfilled and then, suddenly, one of us would come clattering back down to earth and find ourselves plunged into yet another disconnected, fearful chapter where the strain of trying, trying and trying some more was simply too much.

Marc and I had both grown up with one other sibling and it felt natural for us to hope that we would one day be a family of four. The desire was there. But our life together just floated on. It always had. There was never a compass. Never any kind of plan or sense of building towards a better future. Maybe my longing for a baby was partly due to the strange way we functioned as a couple. Maybe because it felt so much of the time like we were play-acting. Pretending to be grown-ups and responsible parents but in reality behaving like we were teenagers who didn't have a clue what life was really about and who probably needed their heads banging together.

Work-wise, Marc was still trying to find his way in London – but I wasn't exactly powering ahead in the career stakes either, and so I certainly wasn't making any judgements from the lofty heights of my own professional success. My dreams of a creative career, first as an actress and then a writer, had come to nothing. Instead, the part-time job I'd taken at a London talent agency just before getting pregnant with Jake had become a steady, reliable, welcome anchor in my life. As had the kitchen-table sideline I'd started which involved managing the fan mail for some of the agency's bigger clients. Answering the phone and greeting clients on a busy West End reception alongside stuffing envelopes with signed black-and-white publicity shots from the comfort of home was stress-free, safe and that was what I needed. I showed no ambition to progress and was happy to stay under the radar. When Jake was tiny it was the perfect set-up for a new mum, and once we started trying for a second baby it just didn't seem like the right time to look for something more challenging. Home life seemed to take up so much of my head space and energy that I wasn't left with much more to give.

Does that sound a bit pathetic? It's so easy to look back and think where I might have been if I'd managed things differently, but I guess going down the *shoulda, woulda, coulda* road is futile. The fact is, we were two bright, capable, healthy adults, neither of whom was anywhere near fulfilling our potential. And, if I'm honest, I took comfort in the friendly faces at work and the low stress, not to mention the much-needed regular income. I counted my blessings that one of us had something steady and secure, and all in all it suited me just fine.

I've always had this theory that Marc should have been my first love. I would have happily let him break my heart at nineteen or twenty. We would have had one, maybe two years together of beautiful madness and thanks to him I would have blossomed from the painfully shy teenager I was into a confident and strong young woman. My first love – a sexy, electrifying Parisian. I could have handled that. We could have avoided most of the trauma and just had the joy. Bypassed the majority of the pain and allowed all the good stuff to flourish. If we'd been young and just starting out, finding our way and not looking too far ahead, it might have been okay – with nothing more to argue about than the odd flash of misplaced jealousy or the occasional passionate French-English cultural misunderstanding. And then after our allotted time together, in a scene from our very own elongated version of *Before Sunrise*, we would have reluctantly but mutually broken up and left each other with nothing but poignantly beautiful memories. We would have met in a bar somewhere on the South Bank and he would have held my hands while I cried into my coffee. And as we said our final goodbyes, Marc would have gently kissed the top of my head and wiped the tears from my face before turning to walk away.

I must go, Emma Blue, he would say, turning back one last time to stroke my face and hold me close. *I need to be in Paris now. You understand, mon amour? I need to go home.*

And he'd be gone, disappearing into the crowds and away from me. Forever. Waterloo Station to Paris, Gare du Nord. It would have hurt but it would have been a sweet, sweet sorrow because I would have always been his *Emma Blue* from Battersea and he would have always been my sexy French boy with the crinkly-eyed smile. Wouldn't that have been wonderful? Our love could have stayed intact. Instead, it turned to poison.

Because, as we know, life is not a movie. And maybe, on balance, it's no bad thing, because if that had been our story then there would have been no Jake – and that is simply unthinkable. How could there be a world without our boy Jake? And there definitely wouldn't have been our Ella or our Louis or our hide-and-seek boy, Theo. They simply wouldn't exist.

So, that night before the crucial egg transfer, I found myself lying in bed alone with a movie of the last three and a half years running through my head. The decision to start trying for a baby – so naive and expectant. The excitement that quickly turned to disappointment, then frustration, then fear. The obsession that turned everything grey and blocked out the sun. The yearning. The lovemaking that turned into functional sex. The three devastating, early losses that left cracks in our hearts.

I set the alarm and made yet another desperate plea to the universe.

Be careful what you wish for had never been more apt.

chapter six
and then there were three

Marc, Jake and I got the bus to Fulham. It was August, the sun was shining and it was the day of the twenty-week scan. Fiona was away on holiday and I'd promised to call her as soon as we'd been seen. I'd been having regular scans since finding out that the IVF had worked, so today, as important as it was, didn't feel like anything to worry about. It actually felt pretty routine. The *routine* scan of our twins. The twins we were told we were having. Twin One and Twin Two. A boy and a girl.

I was giddy and I think Marc was too, on that day at least. It changed all the time. One minute we'd be happily bickering about baby names and the next the shutters would come down and the black clouds would descend.

'What are we going to do, Emma? What are we going to do?'

The news that there were two heartbeats, two growing babies had filled us both with a feeling of mild panic, but there was also a degree of excitement. Jake was ecstatic and I just kept telling myself that we'd cope. I'd finally be able to move on from the obsession that had dominated our lives for so long. Together we would rise to the adventure and everything would work out. It was overwhelming but doable.

I think, mostly, that when Marc and I were with Jakey, we were happy. I'd never known a child so full of sunshine. Joyous company, holding both our hands and chatting nonstop as we took the bus over Battersea Bridge and along the King's Road towards Chelsea and Westminster Hospital.

Twenty weeks! After three miscarriages and so many unwanted periods, it really was a miracle. Only four weeks to go until the babies were viable, meaning they'd have a good chance of survival even if they were born early. Another month of tensing up every time I needed the loo, nervously checking the tissue for signs of a bleed. Nearly there, we were nearly there and on this particular day, that felt amazing.

Because of the catastrophe that followed Jake's birth and the whole flesh-eating bug fiasco, the hospital had promised us focused care. So when our time came to be seen it was the consultant obstetrician who was performing the scan, not a radiographer. He wasn't going to win any personality awards but I knew he was excellent at his job and he got straight down to work, squirting cold jelly on my belly and tapping away at the ultrasound machine that beeped reassuringly to my right.

Marc and Jake stood by the door next to a big screen, waiting with bated breath to see our babies appear looking more real than ever.

Jake's face must have been aching, he was smiling so much. Marc looked nervous but excited. We could do this. We could rise up to the challenge of two babies.

Grey, shadowy, grainy shapes appeared on the flickering screen. Arms, legs, who knew? Nobody spoke.

Ah yes, there was Twin One.

Minutes passed.

And look – Twin Two.

Then the consultant confirmed what he'd predicted eight weeks earlier that yes, Twin One was a girl and Twin Two a boy.

Marvellous. Perfect!

Silence.

Marc held Jake's hand tightly. I looked over at them both, happy, relieved. What a milestone to have reached. Silence still.

And then.

'Was this IVF?'

I didn't really understand his question. He knew it was. Had he forgotten?

'Yes, yes it was.' My eyes darted over to Marc.

Another silence.

'How many embryos did they put back in?'

'Er... two.'

The consultant knew that, surely? Why was he asking these stupid questions? He'd scanned me every few weeks for the last three months. He knew as much as we did about the pregnancy and the two babies that had taken hold. The girl and the boy we would eventually name Ella and Louis.

The silence was ridiculous.

The consultant carried on swishing and swirling the strobe on my stomach. The images on screen made no sense; they were just endless shapes and shadows, unidentifiable apart from the occasional glance of a melted face with a barely formed nose and strangely contoured, wobbly lined cheeks.

I could feel myself tensing up, irritated. All these silences and stupid bloody questions. I had to say something.

'Is everything alright?'

'I think there's a third one in there.'

Everything stopped.

Everything in that moment stopped. Everything except Jake.

'What is it, Mummy?' His little bespectacled, Harry Potter face was suddenly etched with concern. 'What's happening? Are the babies okay?'

I looked at Marc before I answered. He looked back. Fuck, fuck, fuck. What? What did he say? What the fuck did he just say?

'Mummy?!'

'I think there's another baby, darling,' I replied in as bright and upbeat a tone as I could muster.

Marc was silent. I was silent. The consultant was silent.

Jake punched the air like a mini Wayne Rooney.

'*YEEESSSS!*' he cried, his face alight with delight and disbelief.

Nooooooo! cried Marc and I internally — a silent, slow-motion scream.

Later on, when I finally spoke to Fiona, she told me that while reclining on a sun lounger, waiting for my overdue call and wondering why it was taking so long, her partner had laughingly said, 'They've probably found out they're having triplets!'

Ha bloody ha.

But that's the kind of thing that people say, isn't it? The kind of throwaway line that raises a smile or mild guffaw. It's the kind of thing that people say because it's the kind of thing that doesn't happen. Triplets don't just materialise. A third baby doesn't simply appear at a twenty-week, FIVE-MONTH, *ROUTINE* scan. In what universe does a third baby just *appear*, for God's sake? How does Twin One, Twin Two become, in the blink of an eye, Triplet One, Two and Three?

Was this the work of Dr Seuss? Was there some kind of trickery going on?

But it was Theo who'd been hiding. Our beautiful Theo. So ultimately, it was wonderful. It was Theo who as a fourteen-month-old toddler would hide in any nook or cranny he could find. Under tables, in awkward corners. Always hiding. Who, still now, likes to sleep squeezed in amongst every soft toy he owns, curling up in a tiny corner of the bed, foetal and surrounded. Theodore means 'gift from God'. Believer or not, the name was perfect. Theo, our secret, hide-and-seek boy.

'If we'd known we would have offered you a reduction,' said the consultant as I clambered off the couch and we said our sombre goodbyes.

A reduction?

A *reduction?!*

Theo, darling, let me tell you now. You changed everything and you upped the ante more than you might ever realise but, my darling angel boy, you truly are a gift. Our gift. You took our adventure to a whole new level so thank you, my cheeky boy. Thank you.

But seriously. Triplets?!

Now the hell what?

chapter seven
the terrifying return home

Those first few days, weeks and months after the babies were born were simply awful. No happy memories of that time. None, nada, nothing. Honestly, I just can't think of a single one. How heart-breaking is that? What a miserable admission. How angry you might quite rightly feel reading this as someone in the middle of fertility treatment. What a bloody tragedy. I'd done it, we'd done it, our babies were here and all we had was the biggest mess ever.

Marc and I were unravelling at such a great speed in those early days that it swallowed up everything else in its path. All the precious moments lost, etched memories of misery where joy should be. And there should have been so much joy. We should have been shouting from the roof-tops! There should have been a street party with bunting and cake and balloons, a new national bank holiday, there should have been tears of utter joy at the arrival of these three. Marc and I should have been playfully joshing with each other as those early days and weeks passed, exhaustion and elation entwined. Teasing and playfully tutting – pinching ourselves at the madness and miracle of the family we'd created, our love so much deeper for how far we'd come.

From the miracle of their tiny fingers to the doll-sized clothes they wore – they were here! They were mighty, they were powerful and God, how they roared. They were thriving. Triplets. Our triplet babies. Each identified only by numbers on my hospital notes until they burst into the world on a freezing cold Wednesday morning in December 2009.

Born at 11.09 a.m., Triplet One – weighing in at 1.9 kg – big sister, Ella. With blue eyes that quickly turned to gold and a scream that sent the birds squawking from the chimney tops, she made her mark from the start. Louis, vulnerable Louis, Triplet Two, was born at 11.10 a.m. with an anxious, worried gaze and a chest that rattled painfully with each breath. Weighing not quite 1.8 kg, he was so tiny, so fragile and he appeared with not just the weight of the world on his shoulders but also a strawberry birthmark. Quite clearly a very considerate gift from Mother Nature to help us along because honestly, really, how the hell would we *ever* be able to tell the difference between him and… oh, Theo. My baby Theo. Our little 1.7 kg secret surprise. He was pulled out of his cosy corner, his secret spot, into the world at 11.11 a.m. – Triplet Three.

On the night before New Year's Eve, after three weeks spent in the neonatal intensive care unit, the babies were finally considered to be of a healthy enough weight to come home. Easier said than done. Just getting them out of the hospital was a military exercise. It was bitterly cold and I'd struggled to find warm baby body suits small enough to fit. They looked heart-meltingly ridiculous. Tiny little things, their arms stretched out to the sides like mini Michelin men all lined up in a row, strapped into three car seats, ready for the off. I'd been given a family room to sleep in for the last couple of nights to 'practise' being in sole charge without the constant monitoring of the nurses, a rehearsal for how life at home would be. I gathered up bottles, formula, nappies, cotton wool, vitamin K drops, antibacterial hand gel and all the other paraphernalia that their very survival seemed to depend upon and tried to silence the whirring noise in my brain as we prepared to be sent on our way.

Marc had arrived on the fifth floor of the hospital with Jake and my friend Becca who, as the owner of a seven-seater and more importantly a much-needed calm presence, had been selected as the designated chauffeur for this special trip. Marc didn't drive and upgrading our laughable two-door Fiat Punto to something more suitable was another thing on the ever-growing '*shit, we're having three babies, what the hell are we going to do?*' list.

'We're here if you need us,' the staff nurse said in a mildly reassuring way as we slowly made our departure, Marc, Becca and I each carrying a baby to a car seat. It was sweet of her to say it but we all knew the truth. This was it. We were about to step out into the big, wide, scary world on our own as parents of triplets. It was our job to keep them alive, keep them well, nurture and love them. They were our responsibility for evermore. It was too huge, simply too enormous to comprehend.

After what seemed like an age spent down in the dark, damp, underground hospital car park trying to get the car seats squeezed safely in and find room for Jake to sit, we set off. Becca drove us through the streets of Fulham, over the bridge to Battersea and towards home, and apart from Jake's excited chirruping and the odd gurgle from one of the babies, we were silent. Marc and I must have looked like two rabbits in the headlights, only occasionally catching each other's eye. We were so awkward around each other now. The support, safety and warm bosom of the hospital and its incredible team of NICU nurses was gone and there was no going back. We were driving towards our new reality with no idea how it would unfold, and all I knew was that I wanted the journey to go on for ever, so daunting was the prospect of our first night together as a family of six with this strange, broken set-up.

The roads were quiet; it was that funny time between Christmas and New Year where everything is in a kind of limbo. That time when London is quiet but fairy lights still adorn every window, the pubs are half empty as revellers catch their breath and prepare for the biggest night of the year, and everyone you pass looks weary, bewildered and ever so slightly in need of detoxification.

Becca managed to find a parking space right outside the flat, a rare and precious thing indeed. I climbed nervously out of the car and glanced up at the light in the living-room window. This is it then, I thought. Here we go. We all paused outside the front door, fumbling for keys, trying not to trip over car seats, babies, babies everywhere – I still didn't quite understand how they'd got here. Jake was beside himself with big brotherly pride and burst into the grubby communal hall and up the stairs as fast as his little legs could go. Marc was smiling and looked happy to have the babies home at last. Was it just me then? Was I the only one feeling absolutely terrified? Was I the only one with no idea how we, how I was going to cope? Finally up the stairs onto the landing outside the flat and then inside and up another flight into the living room where we deposited the babies down onto the floor, still in their ridiculous coats and still strapped into their car seats. We were out of breath. Those bloody stairs.

Marc, Jake, Becca and I stared down at Ella, Louis and Theo. We were all silent for a moment. Three sets of big, baby-blue eyes stared back at us and I honestly wonder, if they could have talked, what our babies would have said. *Get a grip,* probably. *We're here and you'd better get used to it. You wanted us, you got us, so pull yourselves together and grow up.* Then Louis started to cry and the moment was broken. Jake flopped down on the sofa with the remote control, Becca made a polite exit and Marc went downstairs to put the kettle on. And, just like that, the babies were home. I stared at them all, paralysed, exhausted, petrified. I felt useless and not fit for the job that lay ahead. And it really did feel like a job.

I would have given anything to simply be consumed by life with three tiny babies, with all the craziness that entailed. The colic, reflux, their tiny digestive systems finding their way. I was ready to change thirty nappies a day, to prepare twenty-four bottles of formula because that would have been all. I'd waited so long for this time, even if the most I'd hoped for was a third of what I'd got. As unprepared as I was to look after three babies, I would have given anything for that to be my only challenge. To immerse myself fully in my new life as a multiple mummy. That's what they deserved, these three. They deserved my full attention.

Instead they got a shell. A mother present in body but completely absent in mind.

chapter eight
surely not.
i mean, really?

I'll probably never know if it was having IVF that changed the lump. Or the incredibly high hormone levels brought on by a multiple pregnancy. Or the stress. Maybe it was the stress. Everyone who loved me thought it was the stress. 'You're going to get ill,' Dad would say on an almost daily basis as drama followed drama and life became more like a soap opera than I could believe. Stress, hormones, whatever. All I know is that, at some point, the lump changed. I couldn't tell you when. Can't pinpoint the exact moment when I noticed that the small, pea-sized, supposedly innocent little lump I'd had for years had disappeared and instead, in its place, was something that would later be described to me as a mass.

I only remember the odd feeling as I lay on my tummy in bed, trying to sleep. The strange feeling that I was lying on *something*. I had no idea as I shifted around, trying to get comfortable in the double bed that I now shared only with the babies, that I was lying on a five-centimetre tumour. I was skinny at this point and I'm not naturally skinny. I was thin. I was wired, sleep-deprived and spun out. I had no appetite. Living on chocolate biscuits and endless cups of tea as the days and nights rolled past and the nervous energy somehow kept me standing. Surviving on pockets of sleep that normally lasted no more than thirty minutes.

The babies barely slept. They were tiny, their tummies tiny, they were hungry all of the time and they barely slept. Did you get that?

They didn't sleep. Marc and I were battered and broken. Our love was broken. We were no more. Jake was our glue, our joy and our light, always in between. It was *Kramer vs. Kramer* except neither of us had left. The agony went on, day after day in our flat at the top of a hundred stairs.

The babies would sit strapped into their baby bouncers in the living room or lying in a row on the floor on a rainbow-coloured padded mat, toy elephants, giraffes and monkeys dangling overhead. There was mess and clutter everywhere. There never seemed to be a moment to clear the decks, to wipe the slate clean and start again. Looking back, our utterly chaotic environment reflected the state of our fractured relationship to perfection. There was no order, no respite from 'doing', no quiet corner to find a fragment of mental or physical peace. Home was a stifling, suffocating space punctuated only by the four perfect souls who just wanted our love. Who only required a calm place to thrive. Who simply needed Mummy and Papa to be okay.

Our babies gurgled and grew while we fell apart.

Please. Please, just go. Please, we can't go on like this.

Just go and we can breathe again. I'm sorry. I'm so sorry. Just go for a short while and we can see. Just go, for now, and let me get strong. Leave me, please, to focus on nothing but the babies and their sore gums. Leave me to manage hospital appointments for Ella's clicky hip and Louis' weak chest and let me please have one part of my brain unencumbered for Jake's homework and to make sure we've got enough nappies and baby wipes and formula for the next twenty-four hours. Never thinking beyond the next twenty-four hours. Marking each day and night in new nappies. We can't do this together now. Surely you can see that? Maybe soon but not now. Not like this. Please, for us, for them, just go.

And so, Marc finally made plans to leave. Slow plans. The slowest plans that had ever been made in the history of plans. The minutes and the days and the weeks ticked by and the babies grew and so did the lump. The lump that had changed to a mass. The mass that was cancer. The cancer that was working its way slowly but surely towards the lymph nodes under my arm.

Sure enough, just as the pile of bin liners grew at the top of the stairs, full of shirts and T-shirts and mismatched socks, another lump appeared. At 3 a.m. one morning as Marc slept on the sofa in the living room and as Ella lay awake on my lap in bed and Theo slept to my left and Louis grizzled from his Moses basket to my right, my fingers stumbled upon a new, marble-sized lump under my arm and the world got even darker.

I did nothing for a while. I didn't take action on this lump that could only mean one thing. The penny dropped, the light bulb came on and it was so fucking bright. Of course. Lumps under arms equal lymph nodes. Lumps equal lymph nodes. Lumps. Lymph nodes. Round and round in my head as I changed nappies and kissed the babies' soft cheeks. Yep, it's still there, as I tried to understand Jake's maths homework while debating whether to tackle the stairs that day for some fresh air. Definitely still there as I sat staring straight ahead as the shouting got louder. I did nothing because I was too busy avoiding trouble. I did nothing because surely life couldn't be that unfair? Maybe I did nothing because I knew, deep down, what lay ahead and I knew that he needed to be gone before I could face it.

And finally, the babies now six months old, Marc began the agonisingly slow process of actually moving out. Going back and forth on the 319 bus between home and a rental flat in Streatham, carrying the black bin liners, bags for life and the odd hold-all full of stuff – God knows what. I would look on nervously from the landing as he disappeared down the stairs and out of the front door, muttering under his breath as an overflowing bag slipped from his grasp and pausing to gather himself before marching down the road towards the bus stop. I would stare after him while holding one or two of the babies in my arms and moving from foot to foot, circling a tiny back in that rhythmic unconscious way that parents do. He would return about an hour and twenty minutes later, empty-handed and ready to bag up the next chapter of his history with me, with Jake, with us. The chapter with our babies not even started.

He finally left on a Monday morning in May and so, on that same day, I called the doctor's surgery.

'I've got a lump,' I said calmly. 'But I'm sure it's nothing.' Denial firmly embedded.

'Friday, half past nine,' said the receptionist and put down the phone. Friday it is then.

'It can't be cancer, can it?' I said to Mel over the phone, both of us almost laughing at such a ludicrous thought. 'The universe couldn't be that cruel, surely?'

chapter nine
black friday

Friday 28 May 2010

Is there a better way to ruin a potentially pleasant bank holiday weekend than by having an emergency appointment with a breast cancer surgeon? Because that's when the cancer ball started rolling – on the Friday morning before what should have been a delicious, long, spring weekend. The GP's bog-standard *we'll refer you to the hospitals' breast unit for a mammogram, you should hear from them within a fortnight* approach did not cut the mustard at all and it felt simply intolerable to sit back and wait for fourteen days when I pretty much knew with every fibre of my being that there was definitely something wrong.

It was like a bad dream and I hadn't even had a diagnosis. I can't remember who looked after the babies that afternoon when Dad and I drove to Parkside Hospital in Wimbledon to see a consultant called Mr Sharma who'd kindly agreed to fit us in for an emergency private appointment before his afternoon clinic began. I can't remember who picked up Jake from school and what they said to him to explain where his mummy was. It's a blur like so much of that time. It was and it still is. Balancing paralysing fear with the practicalities of parenting left me on some weird kind of autopilot which I think remains to this day.

'Mummy's got an appointment.'

That's what Jake would have been told. *An appointment.* A euphemism used over the last seven years for so many things. He never asked for what, he barely does now, aged fourteen. A bit like my approach – don't ask questions. If you need to know, you'll know.

I liked Mr Sharma instantly, liked his energy – if that's not too annoying a thing to say. He was warm and sincere but professional. All very low-key. After examining my boobs he asked if I'd had any other kind of symptoms.

'Like what?' I asked.

'I'm not going to tell you,' he said. 'The brain is very powerful.'

Nope, I thought. No other symptoms.

Oh, but hang on. What about the dimpling and puckering I'd noticed? Was that something to mention? Something to draw his attention to?

I'd been sitting in the local beauty salon a couple of days earlier waiting for a leg wax (not realising it would be the last one I would need for a good while to come). I reached for the nearest magazine, grateful for thirty minutes of downtime, and glanced at the cover.

One of the headlines immediately caught my eye.

Brave Bernie's Cancer Battle. Unlike the me of now who will go out of her way to avoid any kind of cancer story, I searched for the right page and began speed-reading the article.

Bernie Nolan – one of the all-singing and apparently always-in-the-mood-for-dancing sisters from the Irish band, the Nolan Sisters, had just been diagnosed with breast cancer. It was a sensitively written but predictable piece with glossy pictures of Bernie looking lovely but pale, wan and staring into the middle distance in true *Hello!* mag style. The tone of the piece was clear. She was strong, she would fight and the doctors were optimistic. She was about to embark on chemotherapy to shrink her large tumour and then she would have a mastectomy.

When did you first notice something was wrong, Bernie?

There was a dimpling, a puckering in the skin on my breast.

That was enough for me. I felt sick. I decided not to read any more. I decided to pick up *Heat* magazine instead and immerse myself in which celebrity was being publicly humiliated for having cellulite and then read about the hotly anticipated *Sex and the City* movie. That was better.

Phew. Let's not read about dimples and puckering, Em. It didn't feel good, did it? It didn't feel good when that shiver ran down your spine and the hairs on your (soon to be hair-free) arms stood up on end. Nope. It did not feel good at all when your stomach flipped over and your mouth went dry.

Dimples, puckering. No. No. No. Let's not go there. Let's not think about that.

'Emma, would you like to come through? Isobel is ready for you now.'

The leg wax felt good and for once I barely winced at the pain. I wasn't a wimp like I usually am. A hot leg wax was something mundane and non-threatening. Unlike the dimpling and puckering I could see on my breast every time I looked in the mirror.

Best not look then, eh, Em? Best not look.

Mr Sharma dealt with things practically.

'So, seeing as you're here, why don't we pop you along for a mammogram? And then, if it's convenient for you, if you're able to come back at 5 p.m. today we can fit you in for an ultrasound.'

'OK, thanks. Yes that's great.'

Which of course, it wasn't.

'And then –'

Oh God, he wasn't finished.

'And then, if we think it might be necessary, we might decide to perform a biopsy.' Wow. Busy afternoon all of a sudden.

Dad and I found somewhere to have lunch between appointments. I say lunch. Neither of us ate. Cappuccino for dad and a pot of tea for me.

Dad and his partner Ro were due to fly to France on Tuesday the following week but Dad was adamant.

'I'm not going until this is sorted out. I can't go not knowing. You're going to be fine though, my darling. It's all going to be fine.'

The minutes dragged, we wandered around Wimbledon Village and then made our way back to Parkside in time for the ultrasound.

I remember lying there and the room being quite full. I remember the atmosphere being very sombre. I remember the radiographer spending a lot of time on my right breast. Stopping and starting, pressing buttons, measuring. Measuring what?

I remember knowing that what they were seeing was bad but of course, at that point, nothing was said.

Biopsy time. Yay. The long, thin needle puncturing my – yep, gotta say it – puckered skin. It didn't hurt but tears slid down the side of my face as I lay there. I remember my ears feeling wet.

A nurse held my hand. What did she look like? Maybe she was blonde. That's right, I think she had blonde, shoulder-length hair. It doesn't matter. It didn't matter what she looked like. She was lovely and squeezed my hand really tight.

'What about my babies?' I said, crying silently and looking up and desperately searching her face for some kind of reassurance.

What about my babies?

Biopsy bandage in place, I went back into the waiting room and sat back down next to Dad but within minutes Mr Sharma called us back into his office.

'So, the biopsy results will be back in on Tuesday. I'll give you my secretary's number and she can –'

Something caught my eye. I looked down at my open bag on the floor and saw my phone flashing. Marc.

Even after all this time, I still had the naive hope that if I ignored his call just once then, rather than then call me twenty-five times in a row, he might realise that I was temporarily unavailable and send me a polite text instead. Something along the lines of: *Hi Emma, hope you're okay. Can you give me a call when you've got a moment? Thanks.*

Silly me.

Again, the phone flashed, this time with a text alert. On silent, but not switched off as it should have been, never switched off – I was never brave enough to take that step and bugger the consequences. Mr Sharma's voice was floating overhead; Dad was looking at me, then looking at him.

'It's Marc,' I said to Dad, my heart thumping, as if he didn't know. We'd had no contact since he'd moved out of the flat on the Monday morning. He didn't know about my GP appointment, he didn't know I'd found a second lump, he didn't know any of it but somehow (because that's how fucked-up my life had become) he'd coincidentally chosen to call right then, in the very fifteen minutes when I most needed him not to.

What do I do? I've got to listen to Mr Sharma, I've got to hear what's being said about next Tuesday, about the results, about what will happen next. I've got to listen and focus and concentrate on this moment. This awful moment of sitting with my wonderful dad opposite this other wonderful man who we've just met whose eyes, gentle smile and body language were telling me that I had cancer.

The texts kept coming.

I answered the phone. Of course I did.

'Marc, please, I can't talk right now. I'm at the doctors, I'm at the hospital.'

I put the phone down and smiled apologetically.

'So sorry, please go on –'

Mr Sharma's face flickered with concern but he carried on.

'I'm sorry you've got to wait over the long weekend to know more. Hopefully we can –'

Flashing, flashing. I cracked again. I pressed the green button on the flashing phone. An innocent phone that had become an object of torture. What I did next was ridiculous. It's almost funny now in retrospect but at the time was pitiful, inappropriate and a bit mad. I threw the phone at the startled Mr Sharma. Not an overarm bowling type throw with intent to injure but a panicked, *take it, take it, you deal with it* type of throw.

'You talk to him. Please, tell him. Tell him I'm here and I can't talk.'

Dad was swearing in the background, beside himself. 'This is fucking ridiculous!'

Mr Sharma took the phone and held it to his ear.

'Hello, who am I speaking to please?'

I could hear Marc's garbled response and it was like something out of an episode of *Fawlty Towers* with Basil Fawlty on the phone to some irate customer and as the viewer all you can hear is nonsensical, speeded-up garbage.

Mr Sharma was, of course, the consummate professional.

'I'm afraid Emma can't speak to you right now. I suggest you let her call you later on when it's more convenient.'

He put the phone down and handed it back to me.

There was an embarrassed silence.

'Goodness,' said Mr Sharma, looking genuinely horrified.

'I'm sorry,' I said feebly. 'It's my ex-partner, it's a nightmare, it's – I'm so sorry.'

Dad leapt in, never able to miss an opportunity to launch into a tirade of fury and frustration at the farcical situation I was in.

'This is crazy! I'm sick to death of it.'

I started crying, again.

'Look at her! Look at the state she's in.'

Mr Sharma chose his words carefully, 'It certainly does seem like there needs to be some kind of... er... enforcement or intervention.'

His words rang in my ears for a long time to come and Dad would, on a regular basis, quote our new friend.

'Even er, Mr er... Sharm, what's his name?'

'Mr Sharma, Dad.'

'Mr Sharma bloody said it. Something needs to be done, once and for all.'

And he was right, it did and eventually it was. But it wouldn't happen yet.

And so, the last 'appointment' of the day drew to a close. It was time to head home, put a brave face on and switch back into mum mode. Perfect. Just in time for a long, sunny, torturous, agonising bank holiday weekend.

Back in the car we were halfway from home when it started again. This time I had no excuse but to answer straight away.

I barely got out a whispered hello.

'Where are the children, where's Jake, what's happening? You never call me, I know nothing about what's going on, this is completely crazy, Emma, you can't do this to me, I want to see my children. What is going on? Tell me! You say you're at the doctors, what doctors? You tell me nothing, Emma, it's unbelievable! I try to be nice to you, I just want to see my children and if you don't tell me what's happening, Emma, I will bring the police, I will –'

'I'VE GOT CANCER!' I screamed the words as loudly as I could.

And then I pressed the red button and threw the phone down and Dad was still driving and only swerved the car a little bit as we drove out of Wimbledon and back towards home.

I think, if I'm honest, there was some tiny part of my brain, in amongst all the madness, that was thinking, 'Hmm, this might work. Cancer might do the trick. Surely he has to be reasonable if I'm ill, if I'm dicing with death? Surely, to God.

Jeez. It's a sad, sad day when you have to rely on cancer to try to get the madness to stop. That's how low I'd sunk though. That's how low I'd bloody sunk.

Thankfully, Ella, Louis and Theo were having a nap when we got back home. I'd somehow got it together enough to arrange for Jake to stay at a friend's house, which meant the coast was clear. No fake happy mummy smiles or forced normality required. I could breathe, I could collapse. Until the babies' next feed at least. Dad's partner, Ro, was waiting at the flat along with Emma and they'd done their best to get the babies settled before we got back. Emma was a wonderful local girl who'd appeared like magic just a couple of weeks earlier and had been helping out here and there with the babies. She was calm, capable and it seemed that absolutely nothing fazed her when it came to helping a strung-out, newly single mum with four kids. She'd prepared their next feed and hung up some washing. She'd plumped up the cushions and made things look nice. I wanted things to look nice. I wanted candles and soft lighting and to burn some incense and do the things that always comforted me. She squeezed me tightly as she left, having gone above and beyond. Ro made tea and Fiona and Dad talked.

'What a man, what a bloody wonderful man Mr Sharma is. You're in the best hands, my darling, you're the luckiest girl in the world! He's the best, he'll sort it. We're all here for you, sweetheart.'

I knew I'd hear from Marc again at some point that evening and I was dreading it. It was as though I'd become allergic to him, to us, to what we'd become. You might quite reasonably think that I wouldn't have the energy or space in my brain to think about us on that dark day. You might think that our demise was the least of my problems. But it wasn't, it really wasn't. It had dominated nearly every waking thought for so long and now it had a companion. Cancer and our broken relationship, jostling for space in my mind.

When his name finally flashed up on my phone the chatter instantly stopped and I could feel Dad, Fiona and Ro hold their breaths.

I didn't pick up, which I knew was pointless and simply delaying the inevitable, but that was part of our well-thumbed script and I was playing my part to perfection. Seconds later it rang again and still I didn't move. We all sat in silence. And then, of course, came the texts.

Emma, answer the phone please.

Then another call.

Then a text.

If you don't answer, I come. Answer the phone, Emma. Please.

Another call. The pattern was always the same. Call after call after call. I finally grabbed the phone and something cracked in my core. Sounds came out of my mouth that I didn't recognise.

'*NO!*' I punched my fist on the nearest cushion, over and over again.

'Emma, why are you so cold?'

'I will be like ice from now on. I will be so cold you won't recognise me. ENOUGH.'

I actually said those words. Melodrama had become the norm. Ice, ice baby. The circa-1990 image of Vanilla Ice and his Max Headroom hair came into my head. Marc was silent. Temporarily stunned. I let the phone drop from my hand and sobbed and sobbed.

All the months of misery and pressure and fights and stress and adrenaline and three tiny babies and too many stairs and not knowing how to cope, not knowing how I was going to stay awake for one more minute, not knowing how I was going to get down the stairs, down all those fucking stairs and out to the shops just for a loaf of bread without help, lying the babies down in the communal hall one by one, going back up and then down, up and then down, over and over. Smiling at Jake, trying to make it all OK, trying to not let him hear the shouting or see Mummy crying, always crying. Trying to restrict the hell to school hours when he was safely ensconced in a world of hopscotch and spelling tests. We could pretend after 3 p.m. that everything was all right. We could pretend that it was candles and cuddles and cosiness in our beautiful kitchen with our beautiful boy.

I roared and howled and banged my fist into the cushion over and over again and Dad and Fiona looked scared but they held me and Dad cried but was also uplifted that his girl, *his* baby had found her voice — had found, on this dark, dark day, her voice at last. I had said no. Enough. Cancer is here now. I need my friends now and my babies and my family. There is no room anywhere in any of the broken cells in my body for more anger and drama.

Fiona took over, picking the phone up off the floor, putting it to her ear and talking quietly as she walked out of the room. I'd roared and he had heard. Briefly, he had heard.

'OK Emma,' he'd said quietly. 'I am here for you. You are strong. You will be OK. We will be OK.'

No, my soul said. *WE will not be OK. I will be OK. Without you. Somehow. I will be OK.*

And then I cried and cried and cried some more.

I'm sorry, Marc. I'm sorry I wanted another baby so much that it dominated our lives. But I didn't go to the baby shop. I didn't go online and order three babies in a moment of Black Friday madness. I wasn't rubbing my hands together with glee thinking I'd hit the jackpot and bugger the consequences. I didn't know this would happen. I didn't know three babies would come. And it's been so hard. Every day so hard, every minute still, it feels hard, but God, I love these creatures. They are my – they are *our* greatest gift. They are beautiful and precious and defiant and they are loud and they are hard, hard work but I will love them for ever and every day I will try to be better than the day before to make them feel that their arrival was worth it. It's not their fault. None of this is their fault.

And afterwards, just briefly, I felt peace. I felt authentic and true for the first time in months, maybe years. I felt raw. I felt stripped back. Cancer had already started its work of stripping me back. I fell into bed soon after. Slept in Jake's bottom bunk under the protective watch of Fireman Sam and Officer Steele. Dad went home, leaving Fiona and Ro to look after the babies. They would hold the fort just for one night so I could sleep. Bizarrely, I felt all right. And I slept.

chapter ten
did i always know?

Did I somehow always know that I was going to get ill? My fear of death certainly goes way back; in fact I'm not sure I can remember a time when I wasn't terrified of losing someone close.

However, it wasn't my own premature end that I fretted about constantly from as early as I can remember. Instead, it was Dad who was the subject of my gloomiest thoughts all those years ago.

When I was small I did whatever I could to not let him out of my sight, so convinced was I that his demise was imminent. Somewhere along the way, my four-or-five-year-old brain had decided that if I was with him I could keep him alive. I could protect him from freak accidents, sudden heart attacks or strokes, from pretty much any tragedy that might befall him. That's a pretty exhausting way to live for a little girl who should have had not much more on her mind than whether or not Alan, Barry, Colin or Tony from across the road were free to play out. Or what on earth was she going to do when she'd finished reading every Enid Blyton book ever written.

I was hyper vigilant, on red alert, scanning, my antennac always searching for danger where, actually, there was next to none.

When Dad (reluctantly) and Fiona and I (less so) used to go and stay with Grandma and Grandad in the Hebrides, Dad's big thing was fishing. God, the fishing. It gave him hours of pleasure and me hours of extreme anxiety.

There was no escaping it. Every day, regardless of the biting wind, rain and bitter cold, Dad would head out to one of several favourite spots and Fiona and I would accompany him like loyal little lap dogs. It never occurred to us not to follow. We would sit huddled together, bickering or bantering as he precariously teetered on the edge of the rocks, fearless and focused. I don't know quite how I thought I would have been able to leap to his rescue if he were to fall but all I knew was I had to be there. Somehow, if I was there he'd be OK, I could save him. That feeling remained well into adulthood. Always hovering, waiting with bated breath in case the moment ever came when I needed to rescue my dad.

'Point', also known as the Eye Peninsula, was the worst. About an hour's drive away, it was a ferocious, threatening rock face with crashing waves and sheer drops. But the best fish, pollocks, rays, flatties were there and to a fisherman, even an amateur one like Dad, its call could not be ignored. We could see it from Grandma's kitchen window, in the distance, through the mist – taunting us as if to say, 'Come, come to me, if you dare.'

Two or three days after our arrival, we would usually have worked through most of the items on our *things we always do when we're at Grandma and Grandad's* list. Number one was the trip into town where we'd head straight for the Stornoway branch of Woolworths. Fiona and I would be allowed to fill a giant bag of pick 'n' mix that we would consume back at the house in front of endless episodes of *Laurel and Hardy*, *Take the High Road* and *Columbo*. It was so cosy. The fire was always on. The cups of tea and treats were endless and Fiona and I were happy to remain ensconced. The only times we willingly moved were when we'd clamber in the back of the Land Rover and head for the beach where Dad would dig for bait, mealworms and the like.

But there would always, always come a point when Dad would study the sky and then mutter the dreaded words: 'I think I might head out to Point today.'

My heart would sink. I hated the place, was terrified of it. I never forgot the legendary story (or was it an urban myth) of the postman who went missing there and whose body was later found floating face down in the sea. To my young brain it was a haunted spot. Every single time we went I would imagine Dad slipping down into the cruel, black sea, lost forever. The fact is he never so much as lost his footing. He was strong, fit and in his prime, looking like a mixture of Oliver Reed and Anthony Hopkins when both were at their rugged, intense best.

And why was it just Dad that I fixated on? Who I needed to keep safe, to keep alive? Was I simply a spoilt daddy's girl, the apple of his eye, his darling Emsy? I remember my heart breaking when Mum left me at nursery aged three, being pulled into the dusty church hall by a horrible teacher called Jean for whom shooing conflicted parents away was simply part of the job.

'Go Trish, just go, love. She'll be fine.'

I loved Mum then and I love Mum now but it has always been different. My love for Dad was intense and unwavering and for reasons I'm still yet to fully understand, the fear of losing him took root in my psyche probably before I could speak.

And Mum wasn't one of those mums when we were growing up. She wasn't soft and cuddly and her arthritic hands weren't smooth and gentle. They were hands that did dishes but they weren't Fairy Liquid hands and she most certainly was not Nanette Newman. That's who we wanted, Fiona and I. We wanted the fantasy mum, the Enid Blyton mum, the Oxo mum, no, God, wait, even better – *The Railway Children* mum! We wanted Dinah bloody Sheridan. We wanted a permanently calm, never cross and always serene mum.

That mum has never existed, not ever. And thank goodness that we now live in an age where we can be candid about the realities of parenthood. We can admit our failings, be honest about the boring, thankless and quite frankly soul-destroying parts of motherhood. Our mum wasn't just *mum*. She was Trish! Feisty, ballsy, no-bullshit Trish. She had her own dreams and desires but Fiona and I didn't know that back then and even if we had, we probably wouldn't have cared. Because kids, on the whole, are selfish little buggers and we were certainly no exception.

Mum's a no-nonsense New Zealander. A real tough cookie. One of five, her childhood comprised of beatings and boarding school and a crystal-clear understanding that she and her flaxen-haired siblings were all firmly down in the pecking order when it came to love and devotion. Parents Bruce and Zeta were firmly at the top, a united front and possibly more in love with each other than their brood.

In stark contrast, it was good cop/bad cop in our house. Dad was creatively fulfilled, loving (with us) and emotionally consistent. He spoilt us rotten. Mum was frustrated, tough, highly strung and thought nothing of chasing us around the house waving a wooden spoon or screaming at the top of her voice in the street for us to come in and clean up our rooms *this instant* or else we'd be knocked into the middle of next week (however that was supposed to work).

To us kids, it was simple. Dad was the safe haven, the one who lovingly carved and painted us wooden elves and pixies that were so lifelike we used to think we could actually see them breathing. He made us doll's houses and memory boxes and go-carts and took us to coffee bars in Chelsea every Saturday and always, *always* said yes to a second ice cream.

Mum was the one making sure we ate our greens, tidied our rooms and practised our scales and arpeggios on a daily basis when all we wanted to do was play out with the other kids on the street. I get it now, of course I do. Once Jake came along, my appreciation for Mum grew dramatically. She was doing her best and she just showed her love in a very different way from Dad. Unfortunately for her, his way was always going to win.

It certainly can't have been easy having a husband with a wandering eye.

'Your bastard father was engaged to two other women when I met him,' Mum would say through gritted teeth as she put the folded polyester and cotton sheets away in the airing cupboard at the top of the stairs.

'Bloody philanderer,' she'd continue to mumble as she mopped the linoleum floor in the bathroom, her Kiwi accent still as strong and strident as ever.

Dad had always had other women. Fiona, as the eldest, was probably much more aware of it than I was, growing up. We didn't judge it or feel particularly troubled by it, but it must have shaped our view of life and relationships and I certainly have no memories whatsoever of affection or intimacy between my parents.

'You were a bloody miracle, my darling, let me tell you,' Mum would say before I knew the first thing about the birds and the bees. When I was old enough to ask how babies were made she'd answer, 'Ask your father,' almost choking on the words as she ran the carpet sweeper round the house and wiped a damp cloth over the grey Venetian blinds that adorned every window.

I do remember them laughing though. Mum would splutter and snort and Fiona and I would cringe as something other than each other tickled their fancy on Saturday nights after chicken, chips and brandy snaps filled with cream. Often it was the TV. The wonder of 1970's TV: *The Two Ronnies*, Stanley Baxter, Dick Emery or Dad's old theatre mate, Dame Edna. I wish I could remember more of what made them laugh. What made the tension dissipate and brought a lightness, so often lacking, into the house. I wish I had memories of a look of love between them, a moment, a hand on the small on the back, an unexpected kiss on the cheek. It would be wonderful to think that their love contained the ups, downs, soft curves and sharp, jagged edges of what a healthy relationship should be.

Unrequited love, my darlings, it's the purest love there is. That's what Dad taught us as he, Fiona and I sat in the Fulham branch of *Dino's* Italian restaurant every weekend and listened as he recited sonnets and spoke of the agony and ecstasy of longing while we ate chips and drank glasses of Coke through red and white striped straws.

Maybe that explains why my sister and I spent so much of our early years in love with boys and then men who had no intention of loving us back. Maybe that's why we spent the majority of our twenties spending every single Saturday night together in my flat. Eating jacket potatoes and ratatouille followed by a mug of peppermint tea. Listening to Beverley Craven's first album over and over again and talking endlessly about life. *Life*, for God's sake! Talking all the bloody time about what we dreamt of, what we longed for, about the romantic love we both craved. God, I wish I could go back in time, put the ratatouille in the freezer, tip the peppermint tea down the sink, turn Beverley off and get us OUT. 'Stop talking, you two! Get your glad rags on! Hit the town! Go and get what it is you dream of. LIVE!'

But the fact is that we had no template so how could we recognise what a healthy love looked like?

I was about ten and Fiona seventeen when Dad moved out. Mum was only in her mid forties – my age now – but a part of her shut down after he went. The drawbridge went up and her heart was closed for business.

It took a long time for Fiona and me to realise that Mum's love for us was just as real as Dad's. It's just expressed in a vastly different way.

So to the little me, the baby of the family, the 'Emsy' who modelled herself on Tatum O'Neal's character, Addie, in the movie *Paper Moon* by wearing dungarees and keeping her hair short, and who simply wanted to be by her dad's side morning noon and night – to that little me, it was simple. My safety depended on his existence.

Dad is in his mid-eighties now. Still strong, fit and only slightly frail, he's never been seriously unwell or had a hospital stay other than to remove some badly behaved wisdom teeth. There isn't and never has been any medication by his bed, no repeat prescriptions, no hospital appointments, check-ups, scary letters through the door, no blood tests, no scans, nothing. If I'd known when I was young that Dad would always be safe, that he wouldn't ever slip and disappear into the Minch and be lost forever or that the ambulances that zoomed past in the 1970s weren't ever for him, that the trees that fell in the famous gales of '87 wouldn't land on his car, that when he coughed it was just that, a cough and not a sign of incurable lung cancer, that his regular headaches weren't caused by a brain tumour but by too many Bounty bars – would I have been happier? Would I have felt a lightness in my heart? Would I have had a carefree, happier, skipping-in-the-meadows kind of childhood? If I hadn't always felt the weight of the world on my shoulders, way, way before I was told I had cancer… would I be different? Or would I have found something else to fret, worry and obsess about?

'You die a thousand deaths, my darling,' Dad would always say and sometimes still does. And he's right. I have died a thousand deaths. But the majority of them I died way before cancer came along. And that is such a bloody shame.

chapter eleven
where's a superhero when you need one?

I started chemotherapy within a week or two of my diagnosis and in the two or three days leading up to my first dose I was impatient. I just wanted to get on with it. Every minute, every hour without treatment felt dangerous and wrong. A silver elixir. That's how I imagined chemotherapy to be and I wanted it inside me. Now.

I wanted to feel it flowing through my veins and hunting out the cells that had lost their way. Wiping out the bad and leaving only the good. I'm sure they hadn't done it deliberately – poor, broken little things – but I needed them gone. I was sure they understood.

Sparkles and stardust. I imagined chemotherapy to be something like magic. I chose to see it that way. I knew the other perspectives. I was very much aware of the schools of thought that saw it as the cause of future cancers, as a destroyer of the good cells along with the bad. They were probably right and if I was a different me, a braver me, I might have said no. I might have turned away from chemo and towards green juices and vitamin C and oxygen tanks and healing and mountain tops and prayer and trust. But I wasn't a braver me. I was a terrified, fearful, cowering me and I just wanted to get on with it. I wanted that stuff to do its job as quickly as possible and just let me get on with my life.

That didn't mean I wasn't praying. Or drinking green juices or politely nodding when well-meaning loved ones informed me that they'd just read *the most amazing article* about the power of lemons or yet another story of miraculous cures and statistic-defying survival and were emailing it to me *right now*.

In those early days Ro made me the most wonderful rainbow coloured food. Plates of pale pink salmon and crunchy vivid peppers, bowls of red, blue and purple berries were placed in front of me at least twice a day.

'Here, have a green tea while I make you a goji berry smoothie.'

'I'm not hungry, Ro.'

'You need to eat, sweetheart. Just have what you can.'

Or Dad would call from their house round the corner.

'We're on our way round with some soup.'

And they would arrive with the soup and I would sit and wait to be served like the Queen. Dad would even bring his own cutlery for me to use – a silver spoon wrapped in a napkin, his favourite salt and pepper cellars and several small, perfectly cut pieces of bread and butter.

'Eat it all, my darling,' Dad would always say. 'You won't believe what's in it. Ro, tell her what's in the soup.'

And she told me and I listened. Afterwards they would take the dirty plates and bowls and spoons away with them. It felt good to be nourished and taken care of.

I remember reading a book on co-dependency, and there was a bit about a girl with who'd spent her whole life caring for and worrying about other people. She spoke of her cancer diagnosis and how at last it meant that she was finally the one being taken care of. I certainly wasn't some kind of martyr or holy-woman carer but I had spent my entire life worrying. Worrying about loss, loving too much and tying myself in knots always trying to do the right thing in every situation. Caring so much what everyone else thought. If you recognise yourself in this picture, you'll know that it's an exhausting way to live. Cancer, on the other hand, forces you to surrender. I'm sure I felt some kind of sweet relief in those early days. It was finally safe to let myself fall, knowing that the parachute would open. I had an army around me. An army that was prepared to hold me up and carry me through whatever lay ahead. They couldn't make it go away but they could hold me through it. And thank heaven the babies were so tiny. Thank heaven I didn't need to tell four little people that Mummy was sick. Just one. Jake. Oh God.

I prepared for it by going online, obviously. I googled 'how do you tell your child you've got cancer' and up popped a book called *Mummy's Lump*. I ordered it straight away, paying extra for express delivery as I'd decided that time was of the essence. Not because I was about to pop my clogs but because the sooner Jake knew, the sooner we could start to normalise this new life. Nothing had felt normal for so long and that's what I craved more than anything else. We needed it. As a new, broken, family we needed to find a new normal. I had to minimise cancer as much as possible and show Jake that it was business as usual, which of course, in so many ways, it was. Everything at home simply had to carry on.

Spiderman was his latest obsession. Leaving behind the chubby cheeks and squeezable thighs of toddlerhood, Jakey was, predictably, turning his attention to superheroes and baddies. Dolby surround sound and glorious Technicolor now captivated him more than Noddy and his mediocre adventures in Toytown. He was changing, moving into a different phase, which was of course perfectly natural. But there was also no denying that, now Papa had left, his cushioned, cosseted, safe little world had already been badly shaken and so I really needed to get this right.

I don't know what I was expecting as I sat in the kitchen and called him down to join me. I fidgeted nervously as I waited for my pocket-sized Spiderman to appear.

'I'm Black Spiderman today, Mummy,' he piped from the hall. The highly flammable (but genius) two-in-one reversible costume was his outfit of choice yet again. It seemed rather fitting given the circumstances.

'Wow, darling,' I said with a rather feeble fake smile. 'Scary! Come and sit with me, angel, let's have a chat.'

Jake clambered up onto the stool next to me, briefly glancing at the brightly illustrated book that I'd placed oh so casually before him. I took a deep breath and began my spiel, quietly confident in the lines I'd rehearsed.

'So, Jakey,' I began. 'You know how there have been lots of people in the flat over the last few days and lots of our friends have been helping with the babies and Mummy has been going to lots of different appointments?'

My miniature Marvel character had already glazed over and could not have been less interested in the comings and goings that had recently occurred.

'Well, darling' – and this was the bit I knew I'd struggle with – 'Mummy's got a nasty lump and so the doctors are going to give me some really, really strong medicine to make the lump go away.'

'OK, Mummy,' said Jake, clearly uninterested and about to slide off the stool and hunt out the biscuit tin.

'The crazy thing is, Jakey...' I said, gently holding his arm and keeping him where he was. 'The crazy thing is that this really strong medicine that's going to make the lump go away is also going to make Mummy's hair fall out.'

There was a silence.

'All your hair?'

'Yes, angel. I think so.'

'Are you going to be bald like that lady off the telly?'

Ah, Jade Goody. A rather controversial nation's sweetheart. She'd died the year before and I, like many, had found myself gripped by how the tragic last few months of this young mum's life had played out. Jake too, it seems.

I did good. I wanted to fall on the floor and howl but I didn't.

'Yeah, isn't it crazy?!' I grinned in what was probably a rather unhinged way. 'I'm going to look a bit silly for a while but it really doesn't matter because my hair will grow back and the lump will go away and I'll be all better.' Please God, let that be true.

'OK, Mummy,' he said. 'What's for dinner?'

And that was that. Oh to be six years old. Oh to take things at face value and oh to be able to live in the moment so gloriously. Enjoy it while it lasts, Jakey, because once it's gone, it's gone for good. And off he went. Spinning imaginary webs and foraging for sweet biscuits that would make everything all right. Momentarily.

I don't know about great power but I certainly did feel great responsibility as I sat staring at the unopened book. Mummy's lump, eh? I didn't need someone else's words in the end. I just needed to speak to my boy truthfully. Bravely and bluntly. Bald mummy was coming.

Jake, can I borrow your superhero costume, darling?

chapter twelve
who runs the world?

From: *Emma Campbell*
Sent: *03 June 2010 23:05*
To: *Katy, Katherine, Amber, Jo, Dawn, Liz, Eilish, Kerry, Julie, Celia,…*

Subject: *Deep breath…*

Hi girls,

Hope you've all had a good week. I can't really believe I'm having to write this email and I'm sorry to shock you but wanted to let you all know so that I don't have to keep saying it over the next couple of weeks when we meet in the playground or bump into each other at the park. I've got breast cancer. The last few days have been a horrendous, horrible blur of tests etc. and I'm still waiting to find out the exact situation. I will be starting treatment next week and the next six months are obviously going to be very tough. I have got to hold it together for Jake and my gorgeous babies and I know you will all be there if I need you – as you have been time and time again over the last year.

As you can imagine I'm terrified but having seen the consultant today I feel a little bit better. He seemed to think things would be OK and that I could beat it. I hope you understand why I'm putting this in an email – I just wouldn't know what to say to any of you next week if you asked me if I'd had a good half term and I can't face the thought of having to tell people over and over again.

See you all soon.

All my love,

Emma x

It was hard to take in the enormity of what was actually happening and I think on some level I must have shut down. I thought I'd hit rock bottom on so many occasions over the last few months only to be dragged down another step. Honestly, I say that without any deliberate self-pity. It was just fact. I'd got so used to each day feeling like a monumental battle that this latest kick in the shins almost felt par for the course. *Cancer, you say?* I'm sitting here imagining Robert De Niro and that thing he always does where his mouth turns down and he looks completely unimpressed with what he's just seen or heard. *Cancer? Right now? Are you serious?!* I'm sure Bobby would just shake his head. Maybe he'd shrug but I'm pretty sure he'd say nothing. What was there to say? Probably quite a lot, but I'd already run out of words.

Single mother! Triplets! Cancer! I thought about that Oscar Wilde quotation – the only thing worse than being talked about was not being talked about – but I could see that this wasn't necessarily true. I didn't want to be the hot gossip on everyone's lips. Certainly not for the reasons I was about to be. But it was inevitable. *Have you heard? Can you believe it? Poor Emma. Those poor, poor babies. There but for the grace of God, oh and that reminds me, I must book that mammogram.*

In my lowest moments, I felt angry that my misfortune might give others a sense of relief that this was my nightmare and not theirs. Maybe angry is the wrong word. Resentful. I never, ever thought *why me?* I really didn't. But I did feel intense envy that people who meant well and who had nothing but love in their hearts might hear my news and feel a palpable relief that they weren't in my shoes. I didn't want to be pitied any more. I didn't want to be the focus. I just wanted to feel normal again, to blend into the background and to be allowed the privilege of getting on with my life like everyone else.

I sent the email to the group of women I met when Jake started nursery. We'd remained a pretty tight bunch ever since, navigating the twists and turns of motherhood together and drinking a hell of a lot of coffee and white wine in the process. My 'school mum' friends. To me they were as essential as Sudocrem and baby wipes – part of my imaginary must-have guide to motherhood. A great group of strong, grounded women who I saw on a daily basis during term time but probably not so much when school was out. Good friends. Easy friends. Friends found at the start of a new chapter in life. We stood together in the playground every morning and afternoon and sat in each other's kitchens on a regular basis putting the world to rights as our children bickered and fought over Lego and snacks. We listened and commiserated with one another about the challenges of motherhood, of trying to keep our relationships on track and of juggling and balancing plates while doing our best not to completely lose ourselves in the process.

These wonderful women had been there for me at so many points over the last few years and never more so than in the last few months of my pregnancy and then when the babies were born. They'd been rallying around long before now. In those fractured months before Marc moved out I would sometimes take sanctuary in Becca's living room on a Saturday morning, the babies lying in a row on the floor as we sat talking on the sofa. Becca's was my go-to house if Marc and I had had yet another overnight argument. Turning up on her doorstep as early as was acceptable with Jake by my side and the babies strapped in their giant, comedy buggy, she welcomed us in with no judgement, kettle on and shoulder ready. God, we were a sorry sight.

In the pre-baby days when things were bad at home, I could just scoop up Jake and go. I could keep out of the way for as long as possible by going to parks, cafés and visiting whichever friend would have us. It was horrible and always felt rather tragic but, somehow, it was manageable. I'd return when it felt like things would have calmed down, we'd eventually kiss and make up and life would carry on – often in a much better way for a while. However, scooping up three babies and making a hasty exit down a million stairs when it all got too much was not remotely manageable. To say I felt trapped in our top-floor flat is an understatement.

I digress. What I suppose I'm saying is that it felt important that I let these wonderful women know about this latest setback and doing it in one fell swoop felt by far the easiest way. So as I pressed send and the email popped into a dozen inboxes across south London it really did feel like I'd exhaled. It was out there now. It was voiced, the story told. Everyone in my world, in Jake's and the babies' world now knew I was ill, and that was a relief. It felt necessary. And what happened next? Well, *that* was really rather amazing.

chapter thirteen
katy, the gang and an attitude of gratitude

So there they sat – a group of women drinking coffee in their favourite post-school-drop-off coffee shop.

All around the same age, mid-thirties to forty. School mum friends.

It was a Monday morning. The first day back after half term. The first day back, which meant that they could focus on work, get the house in order, have a little bit of peace and quiet, breathe in the stillness after a week of noise, mess and full-on family life.

If you were sitting in a quiet corner on your own, maybe reading a newspaper or working on your laptop, you wouldn't look twice at this group of friends. Nothing out of the ordinary: mums chatting, catching up, like mums all over the country.

You probably wouldn't notice that one of the women seems to be holding court. That she's scribbling notes down in a spiral-bound pad. That there seems to be some kind of brainstorming going on. Maybe it's early preparations for the school summer fête? Maybe they're all keen members of the PTA and are working their way through a list of topics and tasks?

Or maybe they're compiling a list of ways they can help a friend of theirs. A friend who isn't very well. Who has three newborn babies and an older boy. A friend who recently became a single mum. A friend who desperately needs friends like these and who is lucky enough to have them.

I had no idea that Katy had called a meeting after receiving my email. I was otherwise engaged. Under normal circumstances I would have been with them, part of the gang. If it had been a regular Monday morning, one from my old life, then it would have been a quick coffee and catch-up before getting on with our respective days.

But my days had changed beyond recognition and there was a point when I couldn't imagine myself doing anything as straight-forward and normal as sitting in a coffee shop with friends ever, ever again. Let alone being the helper and not the helpee.

Helpee. Is that even a word?

It was all her fault. Katy's the one who, as a seasoned mum of four and back when I was simply *Emma, pregnant with triplets* and not *Emma, single mum with newborn triplets and cancer*, told me to say yes to every single offer of help that came my way. I bet she didn't realise she'd be the one doing most of the offering. Well, certainly the organising of the offering, if that makes any sense.

So there was Katy, Katherine, Kerry and Karen. No, these particular K-pals weren't part of some south-London-based Kardashian equivalent but just a handful of the friends who took no time in responding to the news.

Then there was Miles, Sophie, Amber, Jo, Lucy, Lara, Maria, Zazie, Dawn, Julie, Liz – the initials changed but the list went on and on. With each new email or text that came pinging through I felt my spirits lift and my fortunes turn.

I wasn't alone. That was the feeling. I wasn't completely alone.

So, it very quickly became clear that if ever there was a time to say yes to the good things that the universe was offering, it was now.

But was it too soon to think about attempting to say yes to cancer? Even though clearly I didn't really have much choice. I didn't want to accept it but I didn't want to waste precious energy by viewing it as a battle or struggle. I almost wanted to befriend it. Get it on my side. Was there anything to be gained from falling to my knees and beating my chest? The timing felt beyond cruel. It felt malicious and it made absolutely no sense but life hadn't made much sense for such a long time that it felt par for the course really.

Say yes to the universe. What does that actually mean? Accepting everything that life puts in front of us, whether we like it or not? Embracing the bad along with the good? It was one of many mantras I attempted to live by in my twenties when life felt stuck and full of not very much other than a generalised longing for more. God, the self-indulgence. I wish I could go back in time and give myself a good old shake. *For heaven's sake, Emma! You're young; you're lovelier than you realise; you're healthy and strong; your body is working exactly as it should; you're living in a gorgeous flat in a gorgeous part of London; you've never known real loss; you've never known real poverty; you've got a loving family and so many friends. Come on! The world is your oyster. All those self-help books you're reading? Throw them out. All that therapy you're having? You don't need it! These are the good days, sweetheart, these are the days of freedom and fun and adventure. These are the days to live a little, live a lot. See it, feel it, please Em, please just appreciate it.*

But, again, in the words of Mr Wilde himself, youth is wasted on the young. It was certainly bloody wasted on me. I could weep for those lost years. Those years spent hiding like Rapunzel (minus the decent hair) in my beautiful top-floor flat. So creative, so cosy, full of candles and hope but devoid of real life.

I didn't know I was born. Ginger Spice and I had a lot in common. Both fans of writing down our dreams and desires and sticking them somewhere to tick off at a later date. Famously, one of hers was meeting George Michael and clearly there's no denying the girl did good. Mine were predictable and slightly less ambitious. Well, if you count wanting to be the next Madonna as less ambitious. Actually, forget wanting to be the next Madge. I would have settled for a slot as a backing vocalist in a Wham! video. My head was well and truly in the clouds and my feet didn't have a clue which way to turn. But even now I still believe in a lot of the Clinton's-card-style clichés. I still believe that there is a natural timing for things, that often we might look back and see that things worked out and did indeed happen for a reason. I've always believed that life starts at the edge of our comfort zone – but even though those words may be adorned on a fake vintage wooden sign that hangs above the fridge, it doesn't mean I don't spend most of my time wrapped in a sleeping bag and nestled in the darkest corner of that very comfortable place, metaphorically speaking, of course. I've always been extremely good at talking the talk (if I do say so myself) but not so hot on actually walking the walk.

Anyway, back to saying yes in the here and now to help.

'We've come up with a plan,' said Katy. 'Have you got time to talk? What's best, face to face or on the phone?'

She came round to the flat later that afternoon, armed with a notebook and some home-made cake which was a welcome break from the chocolate digestives that constituted breakfast, lunch and most of dinner.

After the babies were born it had become the norm and an unspoken rule that whenever anyone came to visit, be it family, friend or healthcare professional, they would pitch in and help in whatever way was needed. There were always bottles to wash and sterilise or prepare with formula and put in the fridge. There was always, always a pile of teeny tiny dirty babygros to put in the washing machine or clean ones to fold and put away. I say 'put away' – what I actually mean is pile up in a basket in a corner of the bedroom. It was (dis)organised chaos.

On arrival, Katy scanned the living room to see who was in most urgent need of attention, quickly took off her jacket and swooped Ella up. Almost instantly Ella's trademark scare-the-birds-from-the-trees squawk subsided. I was changing Louis's nappy with the speed of an Olympian and Theo – my Mr Happy – was gurgling on the floor clutching at thin air.

'We've had a meeting,' Katy began, Ella now almost calm and about to start snoozing on her left shoulder. 'Everyone is on board; everyone wants to help.'

'Really? OK. Er… thanks. That's amazing.'

'We've all talked about what we can or can't offer and I'm happy to take on the role of organising the rota. The others are going to let me know their availability and then you and I can check in with each other every week and make sure you're getting the help you need.'

'Wow,' I gulped, my eyes welling up with tears of gratitude. 'That sounds great. Thank you.'

'And as chemo progresses and if you start to feel really ropey we can adapt and adjust. What do you think you'll need help with most?'

It was so hard to know quite what lay ahead. I barely knew what chemotherapy was, let alone how it was going to make me feel. Would I be bald, bedbound and throwing up into a bucket for the next six months? Would I be a danger to the children if I was left alone with them? How could I possibly know how I was going to feel a month or so down the line?

Katy struck the perfect balance between sensitivity and practicality.

'Well, this is what some of the others have said they can do. Celia wants to do your laundry each week so if you just bag it up she'll come and get it on a Friday and drop it back to you on a Monday. Katherine wants to be on the list for lifts to and from the hospital as you won't be able to drive and Liz has put her name down to walk the babies. They need fresh air and you might not be well enough to do it.'

Katy paused for a moment; she could see I was struggling. Her lovely face broke into a smile but there were tears in her eyes.

'Thank you,' I mumbled, looking at the floor and feeling totally overwhelmed and undeserving of this amount of attention and fuss.

'We should be thanking you,' she said, clearly trying to lighten the mood. 'You're bringing us all together. What an amazing community we live in!'

She was right. I'd always known that but now it felt even clearer. So much friendship, so much support, woman to woman, mum to mum.

Even though I hadn't seen much of the 'gang' recently, I could feel what was going on. I'd missed so many gatherings, so much of the fun that kept us all going. The early-evening glass of wine while the kids were playing, the coffee mornings and chat, the book club nights that were anything but nights spent talking about books. I'd been off air for a while but I could feel the activity, the connections and the love. And it wasn't just in SW11. The word was spreading and friends from all areas of my life were coming together.

Ali from the gym called.

'We're praying for you at church,' she said. 'People want to help. Can I give Becky your number?'

I had no idea who the hell Becky was but I said yes.

Everyone I spoke to said the same thing.

'We've got to do something, Emma. We've got to find a way to get you some proper help. How are you going to pay for childcare?'

I didn't know the answers to so many questions and certainly not that one. Finances, money – it was all one big mess. Dad was helping as he always had in times of crisis but I hated being so dependent and had no idea how I was going to manage in the long term.

I wasn't part of the maternity nurse brigade that so many of my neighbours and friends belonged to. Paying for round-the-clock or even full-time help simply wasn't an option.

Sleep. Rest. Everyone was obsessed with me resting and the subject kept coming back round to different ways of funding childcare, night-time care in particular.

The night-time feeding routine for Ella, Louis and Theo was something that had to be seen to be believed. Three babies, three-hourly feeds with each feed taking up to two and half hours. It was – how can I put it? – intense to say the least. The babies slept in my room, their Moses baskets surrounding the bed. Ella would be at the foot of the bed, Theo in the middle and Louis to my immediate right. I would stagger upstairs at bedtime, carefully carrying a tray that held eighteen bottles of formula. I looked like Mrs Overall from *Acorn Antiques*. Julie Walters would have been proud. I would place the tray carefully down on the floor alongside a changing mat, pile of nappies, a packet of baby wipes, spare dummies, Infacol for their reflux and teething granules for their sore gums. It was imperative that I had everything I might possibly need for the night ahead. The thought of having to go downstairs, down those cold wrought-iron stairs into the kitchen was just too much to bear. The thought of even getting out of bed was agony. I'd become adept at changing, wiping, feeding, burping and mopping all while propped up in what used to be my side of the bed. Anything, I'd do anything to simplify, to streamline this routine, which, if I'm honest, was hell.

Sleep deprivation is a well-known form of torture but it's incredible how you adapt. Snatching twenty or thirty minutes of sleep here and there was somehow enough to keep me standing. I was just about making it through each day on a few broken hours but that was pre-chemotherapy. My brain simply couldn't engage with trying to imagine how I'd manage to wake up and tend to the babies once the side-effects of treatment kicked in.

But I think everyone around me was worrying about that side of things more than me. Especially my 'mums with young kids' friends. They were all clearly imagining themselves in my shoes and I could feel their own anxiety levels peaking – genuine love and heartbreak mixed with their own very understandable thoughts of *what the... how the...* and *thank God it's not me.*

Without being arrogant enough to imply that I was at the forefront of everyone's mind, I think it's safe to say that my ongoing dramas had been a subject of conversation for an embarrassingly long time.

Trying to conceive.

Miscarriages.

Catastrophic relationship breakdown.

IVF.

Twins.

Triplets.

Separation.
And then,
Cancer.

So there I sat as Katy made notes and Ella slept and Louis grizzled and Theo gurgled. This was step one. I had cancer but I also had so much more than that. I had friends. I had support. There was almost nothing but love coming my way.

Almost.

chapter fourteen
was this our rock bottom?

So what was the point of no return for Marc and me? Out of the many, many horrible episodes, what was the moment that told me there was no going back? Later on it couldn't have been clearer but at the start, in the early months after we separated, it was murky and foggy. It was so incredibly confusing. Good bits, bad bits, nice bits, terrible bits, wonderful bits and horrendous bits. Our relationship had followed a diluted version of that pattern from the start but once we split up it was magnified and the torment and pain on both sides just continued for what felt like many, many lifetimes.

What I don't think Marc realised is that there were few who didn't empathise with how difficult it must have been for him. There was a hell of a lot of sympathy for this man who'd tried to support his girlfriend's longing. Who, when push really came to shove, might have been happy with his boy and his coffee and cigarettes and some cash in the back pocket of his Levi's. He must have been in shock but unfortunately his shock translated into hostility and instead of being on the same team we were locked in a battle.

And I really should be clear about one thing. Marc didn't want us to split up. He didn't do a runner or have an affair. He loved me, loved Jake and loved Ella, Louis and Theo too. Shouldn't that have been enough for a woman who finally got her way, who finally got her babies? For Christ's sake, Emma – shouldn't that have been enough?

Clearly not, and believe me when I say that the *what a bitch* tape played in my head for years. It still whispers to me sometimes. Out of nowhere, when I catch sight of Theo's gorgeous face and the way it glows and shines when he's talking about something that excites him. When I glance up and see Ella looking the spitting image of her beautiful Parisian auntie − my stomach lurches. I won't even go there with Jake. Quite simply, he is a mini Marc from the curve of his legs to the crinkles around his eyes. They are the same in body if not in temperament. How is it that these babies, that Ella, Louis, Theo and Jake don't see their Papa any more?

Where did it all go so spectacularly wrong?

When you break it down, it's actually very simple. Something in me became allergic, properly allergic to living in a permanent state of fight or flight − of conflict.

I could kind of cope with the other stuff. I probably could have carried on putting up with our financial insecurity, staying in our tiny flat, never really feeling like I could take a breather. It might have given me stomach ulcers, high blood pressure and other stress-related conditions but it probably wouldn't have killed me. The kids wouldn't have grown up in a broken home, they might be able to speak a smattering of French and all would have been well. Kind of.

Having the babies raised the stakes. Getting cancer pushed the stakes so high that they disappeared into the clouds. I couldn't take the chance. I couldn't take it for granted any more that my body and spirit and soul would just keep me going. My energy and focus were required elsewhere and some kind of steely NO took over that no amount of wearing down would change.

He did try. But never in the way I needed. He tried because he couldn't, wouldn't give up on us. He couldn't, wouldn't accept that too much damage had been done, that I desperately wanted him to be there for the children but to make *them* his focus, rather than me.

Every single thing that every single other person in my life did for me during that time freed me up to give cancer, motherhood, my best shot. I would regularly be shooed into the bedroom and ordered to lie on the bed for ten minutes while a friend mopped the kitchen floor. Becca would often make Jake tea after school and return him with a full tummy, ready for bed. That freed me up. Jo would call from Asda to see if there was anything I needed, happy to drive by on her way back and drop it off. It freed me. Moments, hours, here and there were lovingly deposited into the Royal Bank of Freedom, the Royal Bank of Recovery. I needed space to heal. To get well. To help the treatment work and for my body and soul to unite.

The irony is that if Marc had set me free when I needed it most, for better or worse, I might just have come back.

chapter fifteen
cake. lots of cake

Amber was my Gwyneth when I was first diagnosed. She was my go-to girl for green juices, smoothies and all things organic. Except I didn't need to go to her, she made it her mission to come to me, passionate about helping me make the right food choices and educating me on what potions and powders might help heal my ailing body.

She was my very first 'mum' friend. We bonded when Jake and her daughter Sienna were weeks old and neither of us knew what the hell we were doing. We were neighbours who became good friends and then ex-neighbours who became even better friends.

Strong, stunning and a dead ringer for Angelina Jolie, Amber has a kind of straightforward honesty that it took me a while to get used to. I wasn't always ready to hear her thoughts on things when we first met. So, in denial about the problems in my relationship and the damage my baby obsession was doing, it might have been easier to choose to spend time with friends who made all the right noises in all the right places. That wasn't Amber's way. Her honesty scared me at the start whereas now it's one of the things I love and appreciate most about her.

In the dark days with Marc, pre-diagnosis and before our official separation I would regularly stumble out of the flat and along the road into her gorgeous house and its Aga-warmed kitchen. I couldn't get the triple buggy in the doorway so I'd leave it wedged inside her front gate and hidden behind the hedge, hoping that no one would pinch it. Though really, why the hell would they? She would help me get the babies inside, we'd prop them up with cushions and rolled-up blankets and then I'd launch into the latest saga.

Whatever sorry tale I had to tell, she would listen intently while making fresh tea and serving up a gluten-free delight. She would take time to give her considered response and when she finally spoke it was always with love and conviction but devoid of melodrama.

'You need to get this sorted, darling. This is serious. You can't go on like this.'

I knew she was right, I *knew* she was right and I knew what I had to do but I couldn't do it, I just couldn't do it.

A few weeks before the babies were born and after months of careful planning and days of endless baking, Amber threw me the most epic baby shower ever. It was incredible. I turned up like a zombie, on autopilot once more. Smiling but spaced out and glassy-eyed. The day before, Marc and I had agreed to separate and I was in a state of relieved, devastated shock, not realising at that point that it would actually be another seven months before the split finally happened and he moved out. There I stood, surrounded by the most mouth-watering display of cakes, puddings and baby gifts and the beaming, happy faces of twenty wonderful friends.

What a day to celebrate! What a day to feel blessed and bountiful and ready to embrace the out-of-this-world adventure that these three babies were going to take me on.

I couldn't eat. Everywhere I looked the girls (and Miles, who wouldn't have missed it for the world) were tucking into slices of cake covered in thick, freshly made frosting, chunks of crumbly shortbread, and bowls of warm, gooey pavlovas. It was 10am! This was breakfast and it was the best, most wonderful, lovingly created breakfast in the world and Amber's kitchen was full to the brim of warmth and support and true friendship. Everyone seemed so excited for me, for the babies' arrival, for what lay ahead.

Hand-made and personalised bobble hats, blankets, wooden toys, vouchers for me to spend in baby departments in whatever way I saw fit. What a happy, excited occasion this was, this should have been. They were coming! Ella, Louis and Theo were on their way! Just weeks to go, this time next month – it was real; D-Day was coming at me faster than a freight train.

'How are you feeling, Em?'

'Oh Em, it's so exciting! It's going to be wonderful, you've done so well!'

How are you feeling, Em? How the hell are you feeling?

How was I feeling? How was I really feeling on that beautiful, bright, cold and crisp November morning? I floated through it. I smiled and chatted and almost joked about what had happened the previous day with Marc. I laughed, made light of my new single-mum status. 'He's going back to France,' I said as the eyes of those around me widened and they stumbled over how to respond.

'It's fine though!' I continued. 'It's fine… we'll be fine. It's good, it's for the best. We couldn't go on like we had. We'll be OK. Maybe things will be calmer now. It's fine. Honestly, it's fine.'

And I walked over to the table and cut myself some cake and I ate all the buttercream icing but left the sponge. Sugar, just give me the sugar, give me a boost, keep me standing, stop me swaying as the walls closed in and the muffled voices got louder.

How did I feel?

I felt broken. But more than that I felt completely and utterly terrified.

So much of my story is about the help I received – help from a million different, wonderful sources. I wish, wish, wish I'd made a list. Kept a log of all of the many touching, beautiful, random acts of kindness. Acts of love. I used to always keep a journal, loved nothing more than purchasing a brand-new notebook and pen and feeling bubbles of excitement at the thought of filling it, scrawling, scribbling down notes, plans and moments. I should have kept a kindness log but I didn't because there was no room in any day or night to sit and process, digest and recall the many good things that were going on alongside the bad. So I barely remember who did what. Who swept in with lovingly cooked meals and who swept out with dirty laundry stuffed into one of those big blue Ikea bags only to return it twenty-four hours later, clean, folded and smelling like a flower-filled meadow.

Which friend was it who turned up at the house one day, cleaned it from top to bottom and left before I returned? Nicky? Ah yes, I think it was Nicky. Thank you, Nicky. I don't think I've seen you since.

And which friend of a friend of a friend was it who heard what was going on and asked for my bank details so she could contribute in some small way? Except it wasn't a small way. It was a substantial way. I don't know that person's name. I might have done, briefly, but it's gone now. Did I even send a thank-you card?

I shudder now when I think of all the unacknowledged deeds. The quick texts of gratitude rather than a call, a hastily written email rather than a card. And no doubt the many, many occasions when I forgot to do anything at all. Shocking. Because that's not me. In normal circumstances I like to think I'm the friend who'll send the card. Who'll remember and acknowledge the good that was shown.

But I know it's all gone in, somewhere. Every single small or grand gesture. Even if I couldn't name them, categorise or alphabetise them in my imaginary journal or log book. You've just got to trust me on this one. It all went in.

chapter sixteen
a house is not a home

Everything happens for a reason, some say. Well, whether we choose to believe that or not, cancer was clearly on a mission to bring everything to a head. *Let's just sort this whole sorry mess out once and for all*, my new pal cancer was saying. *Let's just put a rocket beneath your stuck little world and then try to put the pieces back together, fragment by fragment.*

I'm not gonna lie to you, Em (no idea why cancer now sounds like Nessa from *Gavin and Stacey*). *It'll be painful, it'll be frightening and for a good while you'll think that it's never gonna let up but I promise* (and this is what I prayed that Nessa/cancer was saying) *if you just trust me, I promise there will be some peace up ahead. Just go with it for now, keep your head down and we'll get you there. We'll get you sorted. You and those babies of yours. You and your big boy. I'm here now, and I'm causing absolute fucking mayhem. But I'm sorting things out. OK? Good. Now put the bloody kettle on and get the biscuits out because I'm making myself at home.*

Marc was right to have been concerned about where we would put more than one baby if the IVF was successful. I can now see that I was quite clearly in denial about how important it was to think about the *what ifs* of fertility treatment. But, as you've probably gathered, I wasn't really thinking straight.

Life was measured in cycles. Menstrual cycles. A graph that marked out not only my basal body temperature but also hope, followed by effort, followed by optimism, followed by waiting, followed by crashing disappointment. Over and over again. Rubbing my empty belly, squeezing my barren boobs. *Day 17: did they feel tender? Day 25: is that mild queasiness or just too many Maltesers?* The online bulk-buying of cheap, flimsy ovulation tests, pregnancy tests, sperm-friendly lubricant, vitamins, the putting of life, work, any kind of career on hold. Hypnotherapy, homeopathy, Chinese medicine and acupuncture. The list went on and on. I stopped measuring our lives in days or weeks or happy occasions. It wasn't Wednesday or Thursday or Christmas Day or Jake's birthday, it was Day 1 or Day 12 or, wait for it, Day 31 – three days late! The anticipation would reach feverish levels. *This is it, I've got a feeling, I can just tell, finally it's happened…* And then I'd go to the loo and – *oh*. The tears and black mood would come and I'd crash. Just like that, it was Day 1 again. And on it would go. It eroded our joy.

We did have a vague kind of plan for where we would live if the treatment were to work. Mum had been talking about downsizing for a while and right back at the start of our trying-to-conceive 'journey' she and I would have the occasional chat about doing some kind of house/flat swap. Not that she was living in a mansion or townhouse; it was just a three-bedroomed Victorian semi in Battersea but it was twice the size of our flat and it had the holy grail of holy grails, a third bedroom. But, as exciting as her idea was, there were conditions.

'You'd have to sell your place and buy me somewhere as I couldn't possibly live in your flat. It's so draughty and you're on that awful main road with all the traffic roaring past – I dread to think what the pollution is doing to your lungs. And we'd have to put it all in writing, so it's fair on Fiona. I want a two-bedroomed, ground-floor flat with a garden. And tonnes of storage space, I need storage space. And there's got to be a downstairs loo – God knows how your sister manages without one. What possessed her to buy a house without a downstairs loo?'

She and I looked at a few potential properties at the start of the pregnancy – during the 'we're having twins' phase, the phase that felt just about manageable. Mum got quite giddy as we were shown around high-spec flats near Wandsworth Common by suave, floppy-haired estate agents wearing pink shirts and blue blazers. I'd do my best to keep quiet as we walked from room to room – I knew that it was crucial that she felt that she was making absolutely the right decision for her own life and that the emphasis wasn't all on helping us. But I'd be lying if I said there wasn't a little imp inside me wanting to shout, *This one's fine, Mum! It's got everything you need! Look, it's got two decent bedrooms (though you live alone so really, what's the big deal?). It's got a huge cupboard under the stairs which I know will really float your boat... and look, look Mum! It's got so many cupboards in the kitchen; you know what you're like when it comes to storage space. All those Tupperwares you collect! It's perfect, Mum, just perfect. Don't you think? Come on, let's get a bloody wriggle on, these babies are cooking and things at home are really bad and the walls are closing in at the flat and I can barely make it up the stairs without collapsing and Mum, we really, really need to move things along!*

I didn't say any of those things. Ever. I tried to be decent. I really did try to do the right thing. I promise. To let my elderly mother find her own way and decide when she felt the time was right to start packing up the house she'd lived in for over forty years.

It was around the time that we found out that our two babies were now three that it became clear that Mum was having serious second thoughts about moving house. It was also around the time that things between Marc and I were plunging to a new and utterly miserable all-time low.

I didn't know what to do. I had no idea how to face up to the house swap debacle other than to stutter and stumble, avoid and evade. So I did exactly what I do now with cancer: bury my head in the sand, put my fingers in my ears, sing La-di-da-di-da, turn the music up louder and hope the problem will go away. Marc was getting more edgy by the day. I was getting bigger, more breathless, more lumbering, less able to climb the stairs, more scared of what would happen if Mum really was having serious second thoughts.

One day I suggested a Plan B. I was bright and breezy as I made us coffee and put biscuits onto a plate.

'We could always rent somewhere bigger, darling,' I said tentatively. 'We could always rent out this place and move a bit further out, what do you think? We can't put too much pressure on Mum, sweetheart, we really can't.'

That idea didn't go down well at all. Not at all. I thought it best not to mention it again.

It's funny how some people come into our lives just fleetingly but still manage to leave an enormous mark.

I met Lou through *Tamba*, the Twins and Multiple Birth Association. Both expectant mothers of multiples – she with twins (sensible), me with trips (Jesus) – and both living in Battersea, we were introduced to each other through the charity's 'buddy' scheme for new parents. It's a great idea and a lovely way to connect with someone who might be going through a similar experience and sharing similar concerns.

As I staggered along the road to meet her in a coffee shop on a miserable Tuesday afternoon, my life could not have felt less similar to that of the woman I was about to introduce myself to. It was a bad day, a bad, bad day.

If we could 'see' stress, what it would look like? It certainly felt like poison, which is ironic. Isn't chemotherapy supposed to be the toxic stuff and stress, however off the scale, simply something that we all live with, an accepted part of modern life?

I remember stopping to catch my breath, gasping, always gasping. I leant against a brick wall, just yards from Jake's school and not far from the café were I was meeting this pregnant stranger called Lou.

Marc had called and I was trying to talk to him as I walked. The truth was finally out. I'd told him that Mum was wavering and his reaction was just as I'd feared.

'Marc, please, calm down,' I gasped, breathlessly. 'I'm sorry.

Please. I'll sort it, I'll speak to her. I'll get Dad to speak to her. It'll be okay.'

Finally he hung up and I stood still, heart pounding. The café was on the next corner and God, I really didn't want to be seen in this state.

I looked at my phone – five to two. I had time. I rang Dad. Poor Dad – yet another hysterical phone call from his hysterical daughter.

'Your mother's changed her mind, my darling,' he confirmed quietly, also in on the fact that this day of reckoning had been on the cards for a while now. 'She doesn't want to move. It's too much for her and she wants to stay in the house.'

What could I say? What could I do? For weeks I'd known this was coming. I knew it and I sensed it and my jaw ached with the tension and my head throbbed with the weight of the knowledge that this day would come and that when it did all hell would break lose.

It was her choice, her prerogative. It was her house, for God's sake. She didn't owe it to us and it certainly was not ours to claim. There was no contract, nothing set in stone or signed in blood. It had been a conversation, several conversations over several months that had turned into a vague plan and I had run with it like the desperate woman I was. And then, very quickly, it had became the big, pesticide-free, soil-covered, organic carrot that I dangled in front of Marc as I tried to convince him to give IVF a go.

'It'll be perfect!' I said to him on the day that Mum and I had talked about it just enough to make it feel like a real option.

'Jake can stay at the same school, we'll still have the same support network, we love it round here. It's just like a house swap except she'll have a flat but oh, darling it could work so well!'

Marc didn't take much convincing. Why would he? Who wouldn't want to move out of a perfectly acceptable but cramped two-bedroom top-floor flat into a three-bedroom house with a garden just round the corner? It could all be perfect – a neat and tidy solution and our white picket fence happy ever after.

What on earth made me think that was possible with us as fragile as we clearly were? What was I thinking? That was the whole problem. I wasn't thinking, I was pushing down the concerns, batting them away and stuffing them into a part of my brain that I tried to visit as little as possible. The part called reality. When you want something as much as I wanted a baby you can convince yourself of anything.

I took a few deep breaths, calmed myself and tried to push all this to the back of my mind as I dragged myself into the café. Lou and I greeted each other warmly with a hello hug, our bumps bumping. I liked her immediately. A year or so younger than me, from Northern Ireland, she was open and chatty. Somehow, for the first twenty minutes or so, I managed to fake it. I think I just about managed to come across as normal, i.e. not on the brink of emotional and physical collapse.

We sped through the 'getting to know you' checklist and quickly established that we'd both had our IVF treatment at the same clinic with the same consultant, were both having two boys (though of course I had Missy Ella cooking away too), were both booked into the same hospital under the care of the same team, and were both in complete and utter denial about what looking after more than one newborn baby would involve.

So, job done. We'd connected, we'd 'buddied' up and it was nice.

That's where the similarities ended.

Sat side by side, bumps out for all to see and marvel at, we sipped our tea and once I'd asked Lou every kind of question I could to delay the spotlight being turned on me, the inevitable happened.

'So,' she asked smiling, 'what about you? How's your husband coping with it all?'

'Oh,' I stuttered nervously. 'Er… we're not married. Marc, he's er… well, er… it's all been a bit stressful.'

I started babbling. It all came pouring out. How bad things

were between us, how they were getting worse by the day. How I'd built my 'one more baby' dream on a foundation-less house of cards that had dramatically fallen apart. How I felt so, so guilty for the mess that we were in. How Mum had changed her mind about us moving into her place which of course was up to her but God I don't know what to do, I don't know how we're going to cope or where we're going to live, where are we going to put the babies and we haven't got any savings and I keep saying to him that we can rent somewhere bigger a little further out but I just don't know if that's going to happen. I don't know what we're going to do.

And then silence. When I eventually paused for breath, Lou simply looked stunned.

'Jesus Christ,' she said. 'You poor thing. And here's me sitting here moaning about the decorators not painting the nursery the right shade of blue.'

I didn't feel I deserved to be pitied. I felt weak. I felt like I deserved all of the blame, all of the fury and threats. Weak. That really is the word. My nervous system was under attack. The stress felt like poison. A thick, black, sticky tar. I was drowning in the stuff. I'd presumed that it was my uterus squashed up against my diaphragm and compressing my lungs that stopped me from breathing normally. If only. I think, in fact, I was gasping for air. For relief. I was gasping for peace.

Lou certainly didn't need to feel guilty for talking about the normal challenges of preparing for twins. She had every right to feel concerned that the nursery wouldn't be ready in time or that she might not manage to breastfeed or that her mum wasn't round the corner to help and offer support. Her concerns were normal and completely valid. I would have given anything to be normal like Lou.

That was the one and only time that Lou and I met for coffee but her involvement in my life carried on in the most remarkable way. Random Acts of Kindness doesn't even cut it. Sometimes I would arrive home to find a huge bag of goodies hidden near the front door. DVDs, gorgeous toiletries, a beautiful warm scarf, maybe some unworn designer jumpers she thought I might like. Like? Like?! I was like a kid on Christmas morning as I reached in and discovered one delightful gift after another.

I caught her out one day. A hand-delivered envelope dropped through the letterbox and as I opened the door to see who it might be from, there she was, leaping into her car, clearly hoping not to be spotted.

'Hey! Is this from you? Can you pop in for a coffee?' I called out as she revved up the engine, intent on making a quick getaway.

'Oh hi! Er, yes, it's nothing, just a little something. Got to dash, sorry Em! How are you keeping? You're looking great! Catch up soon, OK?' And she was off.

The envelope contained a gift voucher for a beauty salon in Knightsbridge. Knightsbridge! I did a double-, triple-take at the value. A three-figured amount that would leave my skin with a glow I hadn't seen for decades. The goodie bags continued throughout my treatment and beyond. And then there was the charity tennis match her husband's company organised every year. Would I mind if they raised money for me and the babies this year? 'To help you through, that's all. Is that OK, Em? Would you mind?' Oh, Lou, Jim – thank you. Thank you so much. As we eased ourselves up off the sofa in the café that day, hugged and said a warm goodbye, promising to keep in touch and wishing each other luck, Lou was clearly lost for words – something I would be on many occasions in the coming months thanks to her incredible kindness.

And Mum's house/flat swap idea? It was an act of love, I know that. She adored Jake. She saw my longing and she wanted to help. Of course it came from love. Her intentions were honourable and I couldn't blame her for changing her mind. It just caused one hell of a bloody mess.

chapter seventeen
a matchbox house of dreams

After Marc had moved out and within a couple of days of my diagnosis, the big elephant in the room, the huge lumbering creature who with every giant step shook the floors, walls and put cracks in the ceiling, was finally being dragged into the spotlight.

Finding somewhere else to live for me, Jake and the babies. It was ironic really. This was the very subject that had caused our relationship to finally implode. The toxic issue that triggered so many scenes was now going to be swiftly and neatly resolved within a matter of days.

The current and completely unsustainable daily routine at the flat with the babies went something like this:

- Mid-morning or mid-afternoon, I decide that I need to get out of the flat with the babies to go to the shops, pick Jake up from school or simply give them some fresh air (because they haven't stopped crying for three hours and I'm on the verge of a breakdown). Have immediate second thoughts and wonder if there's a way that I can avoid going out.
- Realise that there isn't.
- Pack bag with anything and everything I might need for our 'jaunt' into the outside world.
- Leave babies alone upstairs while I take the heaviest bag in the world downstairs and leave it by the front door in the grubby communal hall.

- Drag giant, cumbersome triple buggy out of the front door and hump it down the front steps before leaving it inside the gate, hoping it will still be there when I come back down.
- Go all the way back upstairs and pick up one baby and a blanket.
- Take baby downstairs and lie baby down on the blanket in the hall, on the floor.
- Do quick tidy of the many takeaway delivery leaflets that are scattered around and letters addressed to people who moved out years ago.
- 'Run' back upstairs and pick up baby number two (while making half-hearted soothing, lullaby-type noises to crying baby number three who must be able to sense that he or she is about to be temporarily left behind).
- 'Run' back downstairs with baby number two and his or her blanket.
- Lay him or her carefully down on the floor next to baby number one.
- Stumble back upstairs for the final time to collect wailing, abandoned baby number three.
- Stagger back down and, still holding baby number three, go outside to giant buggy that nobody wants to steal and strap baby inside.
- Strap in remaining two babies, shove dummies in their mouths and make silly faces as I lock the front door.
- Realise that I've forgotten something absolutely crucial like baby wipes or purse or bottles and try not to cry.
- Cross my fingers, pray to Jesus that no one will try to steal three babies while I sprint all the way back upstairs like Jessica Ennis to retrieve forgotten item.
- Come back down, gasping for breath and utterly exhausted, still on brink of tears.
- Feel immense relief that no one has stolen babies.
- Realise it was highly unlikely that anyone would.

I probably could have struggled on like that – if I'd had no choice then I would have had to. It was still a home, still a warm, cosy home with beds and running water and nice bits and pieces everywhere. I knew that, compared to many, I was still very fortunate. But cancer came and, like on a two-pence arcade game on Brighton Pier, it was the coin that finally shoved the other teetering coins over the edge. Cancer was the tipping point. Visions of me green round the gills and flailing around after chemo, lucky enough to have offers of help but not well enough to stagger downstairs and answer the door with its broken intercom – it was an absolute no-brainer; I needed to rent somewhere and rent somewhere fast.

Mel, Fiona and Dad took the lead and found a small house for us to look at, about a mile or so away from the flat, near Wandsworth Common.

We arrived, parked up outside and trailed in behind the pointy-shoed and shiny-suited lettings agent. The house had no high ceilings, no interesting features, cornicing or open fireplaces. It was a new build, it was uninspiring but I fell instantly in love. It was empty and clean and neutral and that was all I wanted. A blank space. No clutter, no teetering piles of washing, no drawers half open, cupboards that wouldn't shut, no draughty windows or creaking floorboards. The kitchen was tiny, the bedrooms were tiny – but there were three of them! Three bedrooms! It was more than I'd dared to dream of. I separated from the others and wandered around like Dorothy in Oz. I could breathe here. It was a fresh start; we could be happy here, I could – oh and look! Look. A garden! I burst into tears.

Fiona appeared behind me.

'Em, what is it, sweetheart? What's wrong?'

I fell into her arms.

I'd forgotten. Just for that moment, as I'd imagined going to Argos to buy a cheap plastic swing and thought about Jake splashing around in a paddling pool and the babies eating grass, I'd forgotten.

'What is it darling? Tell me —'

'I forgot I was ill,' I spluttered. 'I walked out here and was so happy and excited that I forgot I had cancer.'

I could tell that Fiona was mouthing to Mel over my shuddering shoulder. Mel discreetly turned away and kept the agent talking for the next few minutes while I composed myself.

As we drove away we were all quiet but all thinking the same thing. This was where I needed to be. This was where my four babies and I needed to be so that I could heal and we could move forward. This would be our happy place. Our safe space. Our new home.

And within about ten days that's what it became. In the days following my first cycle of chemotherapy and as my hair was falling out in handfuls I started frantically packing up the flat ready to move and attempting to leave it in a fit state to rent out. Stuff, so much stuff. A lifetime of *stuff*. When I think back it's a blur. How the hell did we do it? Who helped, who organised viewings for potential tenants, who sugar-soaped the walls and mopped the floors, who emptied the wardrobes and the kitchen cupboards and the drawers of doom with the random wires and batteries and phone chargers and who made sure the kettle was always on and who offered car space and precious weekend hours and strong arms to lift boxes and who entertained the kids while Jake, Ella, Louis, Theo and I moved from one place to another?

They all did. They all helped. All the friends, all the mums, all the women, Dad, Ro, and lovely Miles and friends' husbands and brothers of husbands who came with vans and packed up everything that was left and delivered it safely to our new home. It was a village effort, a postcode effort and there I stood, in the middle of it all – grateful and in awe of the many, many wonderful humans in my life.

Moving day itself was a chemo day for me. Cycle two. I arrived back to find everyone going in and out with boxes and bags and babes in arms and mugs of tea for the heavy lifters and questions immediately being fired at me about where I wanted things to go.

'Anywhere. It's home. We'll sort it out. Thank you, thank you so much.'

Dad was on the front doorstep and as I slowly clambered out of the car feeling the beginnings of the *post-chemo hit with a truck* sensation take over, I could see he was giddy, as high as a flipping kite.

'You're the luckiest girl in the world!'

A tall, dark-haired woman was standing next to him on the doorstep, smiling brightly.

'You've got a doctor living next door! What did you say your name was, my darling?'

He was beside himself. Elated that Nicki – a consultant obstetrician – lived, not actually next door but in the flats on the corner and she'd come by to say hello. As if the close proximity of a woman who dealt with high-risk pregnancies would make me more likely to recover from breast cancer. My wonderful dad: he was so desperate to see me safe and protected. But really, that's what the close already felt like – like an oasis of safety and peace in a world that had become so frightening and rocky.

The second knock at the door came the day after we moved in. There stood Peter, Emma and their children, Charlotte, Pippa, James and toddler Alice – neighbours from number fourteen. Emma was holding a plate of home-made muffins. A touching, thoughtful, welcome-to-the-neighbourhood gift. I stood weeping by Dad's side as he talked nonstop, giving them a potted version of recent events. Jake appeared behind us and said a shy hello to the only boy in the family, James. They were almost exactly the same age. Their friendship was instant and beautifully confirmed what I already knew – that the close was where the five of us were supposed to be.

A leaflet fluttered through the door later on that week. Printed out on a home computer with multicoloured font and a generic image of yellow flowers at the top.

Hello and welcome to the close. We live opposite at number 6. We can see that you've got your hands full so we'd love to offer our help in any way

– babysitting or shopping. If you need anything just ask. Love from John, Jo, Rosa and Lily.

They didn't wait for me to ask. Shortly after, Rosa and Lily knocked on the door with flowers from 'John's garden'. The stunning, abundant, wild front garden that their step-father spent every spare minute cultivating. It was the first thing you saw as you turned into the close. It was my view from the sink in our dated, tiny, uninspiring kitchen.

John isn't here any more. He was diagnosed with cancer a couple of years after my diagnosis. It showed no mercy. But his garden still thrives. Differently of course but, thanks to Jo, it still thrives. It's still John's garden.

Fucking cancer.

Rosa and Lily were thirteen and fifteen when we moved in. Thirteen! Their tender, inexperienced ages meant nothing to me. They were simply more hands, more help. More walks in the park for the babies and more smiling faces for them to lock onto. I just trusted, somehow, that everyone was nice, decent and good. And they were. I had faith that my babies would be safe with whoever held them in their arms. And they were.

chapter eighteen
thanks for the smiles, mark

When it came to losing my hair, the 'waiting' bit was the worst. The stark realisation that once it started falling out it wouldn't stop. How long would it take? Would I wake up one morning and find it all on the pillow and my startled scalp shining brightly like a piece of polished marble?

I remember hearing a story (that, surely to God, can't possibly have been true) that a woman going through chemo went for a ride in an open-topped sports car and ALL her hair flew off in one fell swoop. I mean, really. *Hair last seen flying down the M1?* Surely that can't have happened but it bloody terrified me.

Mine started shedding, as I'd been warned, between the first and second cycle. It started with strands. A few and then, quite quickly, a lot. I quickly purchased a cap to sleep in. A soft, lilac-coloured chemo cap to designed to keep my bald head warm at night but it was also – top tip alert – a very handy way to keep the strands contained. This was a big bonus as Jake had taken to sleeping in my bed every night back then and I didn't want to traumatise him, poor boy.

And then the day came when it really was going, going, going and I just needed it to be gone.

As previously arranged, I gave Becca 'the call'.

It was time.

Becca and her hairdresser husband Tony arrived at the house that same afternoon. It was quite fitting actually as Tony is the proud owner of his own shiny bald head, the perfect man for the job. Jake had been whisked off to Dad's for a few hours and Becca kept a watchful eye on the babies while Tony and I went upstairs.

There was nervous, slightly inane chatter for a minute or two.

There were no tears.

There was a lot of adrenaline.

I sat on a fold-up chair in the middle of the bathroom, towel around my shoulders, and Tony set to work. No nonsense. No faffing.

'Let's just get rid of it, darling,' he said. 'You'll feel so much better afterwards.'

Out came his trusty razor and clippers. It took about two minutes and it was done. It took me a few minutes more to pluck up the courage to take that first look in the mirror and when I did it was just… odd.

Deep breath.

Right then. That was that.

It was almost like a *roll your sleeves up, let's get this show on the road* moment.

No more pussy-footing around. Hair gone: one less thing to think about. It would grow back. I *would* have hair again.

Early the next morning I was on my knees in the living room doing up the poppers on Theo's babygro. I had my lilac cap on. Jake was messing around on the floor next to me, tickling Ella's toes and blowing raspberries on Louis's belly.

Suddenly, he sat up and – quick as a flash and before I had time to stop him – he yanked the cap off. We both shrieked. Jake literally fell backwards in shock. I grabbed it back and quickly pulled it down over my head.

He looked horrified.

I wasn't brave in that moment. I felt angry, embarrassed, exposed. And then I got a grip and pulled myself together. I hoisted my weary body up off the floor and walked into the kitchen to deposit yet another steaming, stinking nappy sack into our permanently overflowing bin.

Hands washed, kettle on, two slices of toast in the toaster.

'Marmite or jam, Jakey?' I called.

'Marmite please, Mummy.'

'Marmite it is, Jake. Sorry to scare you, darling.'

And another busy day had begun.

Who knew being ill could take up so much time? If I wasn't at the hospital then it was business as usual at home. We had a routine to follow. Despite the fact that, pre-triplets, my natural rhythm and approach to motherhood was to take each day as it comes, go with the flow and make it up as I went along, this time around it was different. Dramatically so.

No lie-ins, no lolling around in my pyjamas like a poorly person. The babies would wake up at about six and it was action stations from that moment on. Get up, throw some clothes on (it would be years before I had the luxury of an early morning shower), get the babies out of their cots, change their nappies, wake Jake up, make his breakfast, start washing the bottles from the night feeds, put the first wash of the day on, empty the dishwasher, feed the babies and... hang on. When did I fit in the two-hour feed before leaving to take Jake to school? I must have, somehow, but I'm buggered if I can remember how.

The first phase of the day ended as I locked the front door behind us and started the walk to school with Jake. I can't describe the sense of achievement I felt as we set off on the half-hour trek. I was doing it. I was managing. While so many people around me were desperately worried about whether I could, and one or two seemed to be waiting for me to fail, I was somehow standing upright and putting one foot in front of the other.

No wonder I was skinny. Pushing that bloody triple buggy around. The ABC Mountain Buggy, built for rocky terrain and triplets. It was a dead weight. Ella was in the top, Louis and Theo underneath. I always planned to alternate but somehow, Missy Ella always tended to end up plonked in the top seat like the Queen with the boys down below, two peas in a flipping pod, cheeks popping frantically in and out with their dummies like that baby on *The Simpsons* and Ella sucking on her stinky muslin which was a health hazard all of its own. Breadsticks, mini rice cakes and baby wipes were stashed underneath, anything and everything to keep them content and quiet. Once we'd dropped Jake off I would often stay out as long as possible just so I could breathe. It was summer, mid July and then August. It was hot. My arms and legs would ache and my back would be wet with sweat on the way back home but as physically exhausting as it was, at least the babies were contained and I somehow felt in control for a bit. Once back at home it was a totally different story, Ella rolling one way, Theo the other and Louis arching himself backwards and wailing on the living-room floor. Who did I tend to first? How did I choose? Every day a million dilemmas; my whole life was like a mini, diluted version of *Sophie's Choice*. Oh Meryl, I really do sympathise.

I know we looked a bit of a sight when we were out in public and that's something that hasn't changed but back then – picture it – I was the lady doing her best to rock the cancer look in Asda with, hang on, how many babies?

'Are they twins?'

'No. Triplets.'

'Triplets?! Oh my God. Janice, look – triplets.'

'I've never seen triplets before.'

And then the brazen, straight out with it, who cares that it's none of your business question: 'Were they natural?'

And then, depending on who was doing the interrogating, the response would fall somewhere between: 'They're a blessing from God!' or: 'Christ almighty, love, I've got two and that's enough.'

I always smiled politely even when the *don't worry, sweetheart – at least they'll look after you when you're old* line was spouted. I'd smile politely knowing that, if I chose to, I could floor them with a few short words. I could lay them out.

Will I be here? Will I? Will I be here when my babies are all grown up? Will I get to be that old lady with the beard and the bunions and the worrying signs of dementia? Will I get the luxury of being an inconvenience, the *it's your turn to have Mum this Christmas* problem?

And there was Jake, scooting alongside us, chatting away.

You could see people do a double-take. Scanning us. Hang on, is that… twins, no… one, two, THREE of them? And another one? Oh and God, look, she's not well, poor cow.

An old woman came up to us in Marks and Spencer's once. I was manoeuvring the buggy round the salad aisle and there she was. Tiny. She had a selection of meals-for-one in her basket and her free hand was clenched tight.

'Here you go, darling,' she murmured, and before I knew it she'd pressed five pounds into my hand.

'No, no, I can't! Thank you but please, I can't.'

'Take it, sweetheart, for those poor babies. God bless, my darling. You take care.'

And off she went. Heading towards the sweet aisle for a bag of toffees and some digestive biscuits.

I felt embarrassed but so, so touched. I didn't need five pounds that badly but what a lovely, sweet gesture. I didn't quite know where to look. I paid for my shopping and started the trek home.

How did I look to people? Were my babies and I such a pitiful sight? I wonder what I would have thought if I'd seen us? Would I have looked away, shuddering and thanking God it wasn't me? Would I have smiled sympathetically and then gone about my business? I could tell that we were 'known' in the area. People would look at us in a certain way, either smiling a little too brightly, nervous and unsure, or just downright bloody rudely. Slack-jawed and agog.

Mark Owen from *Take That* used to live nearby and I often spotted him out on Wandsworth Common. He sometimes used to smile and say hello. It gave me a little thrill to keep a look out for a twinkly-eyed pop star on a gloomy, post-chemo Thursday when all I wanted to do was sleep and cry. The hours spent on that common, wandering, twisting and turning. Walking one way and then the other. They're asleep, just keep walking; they're crying, just keep walking. Might bump into someone I know and be able to have a chat, might see Mark Owen, might get a smile. Might get a little mood-enhancing smile from an ex-boyband heartthrob who's now himself a father of three with his own ups and downs and sleepless nights. He was famous for being the Harry Styles of the nineties, the boy with the killer smile, the boy that broke a million hearts, and I was a familiar face in the same postcode for being bald and for pushing a giant buggy with lots of babies strapped inside.

Maybe he looked out for me too. Highly doubtful but you never know. Maybe he used to wander past the café on the common, past the dog-free play area and wonder if he'd see the woman wearing a hat that covered her bald head. The woman pushing the buggy that contained so many babies. The woman that didn't know what the hell had happened to her life and who was just putting one foot in front of the other. Round and round the common. The woman who didn't know what else to do.

We're all the same when it comes down to it.

Living with fame and fortune or drowning in a fiscal fiasco. A painstakingly coiffured head of hair or the barest of scalps. Cancer or no cancer.

We're all the same.

chapter nineteen
note to self: always wear knickers to chemo

I can't tell you much about chemotherapy itself and what the sessions actually involved. I'm never sure if my lack of memory when it comes to details about my illness is due to chemo brain or some kind of coping mechanism – never wanting to know more than the sketchiest details about what was going on. So different to how so many other patients handle things but it's the only way I know.

I can't remember what my drugs were called. I do remember each chemotherapy session taking about three or four hours all in. I remember falling into the deepest of sleeps at various points, head lolling forward, waking up with a jolt to discover that only seven minutes had passed. I remember vials of blood being taken and knowing how crucial the results were but never wanting to know the numbers, the levels, the dreaded tumour *markers*. I remember getting weaker and weaker with each cycle, so weak that by the time I was on cycle number seven I became dangerously ill with neutropenia – the white blood cells (so crucial to fighting infection) wiped out by the brutality of the treatment that was supposed to be saving my life. I remember being admitted into hospital, where I stayed for several days, and not realising how seriously unwell I was as I kicked up a fuss and begged to be allowed to go home to my babies.

'You've got four children, right?' said Professor Ray Powles, Trevor's identical twin, who popped in to see me on his brother's behalf. 'You want to be at their weddings, don't you? See them graduate from university? Let us take care of you then. Let us do our job. OK?'

That put me in my place. He said it with a twinkle in his eye and a soft tone but the message was clear. Pull yourself together, Emma. Accept that this is where you need to be. Let us get you well, get you strong. Keep you strong for your babies.

If I'm honest, I mostly preferred being left alone during chemo sessions. If all was going to plan then it was quite nice to have a few hours to myself with nothing to do. I could have that drug-induced snooze, sit and stare into space while wondering what the hell had happened to my life, have a little weep, all in peace. Nice hot cups of tea, a few biscuits here and there, it wasn't horrendous. The actual chemo sessions themselves were never as bad as the days that followed when the side-effects of nausea, flu-like symptoms and exhaustion – to name but a few – really kicked you in the head with their size twelve steel-toe-capped Dr Martens.

But if certain friends wanted to join me – most likely the ones who I didn't get to see that often, who were visiting and desperate to feel useful in some small way – then of course, their presence was a welcome change from the gloom of my own black thoughts. And there aren't many people I know who are as incredible at lighting up the dark as my friend Jess.

Oh Jessie. My larger-than-life girl, my storyteller, my exclaimer, my 'Em, you're not going to *believe* what's happened!' buddy.

I've known Jess forever. Her big brother Jake and my sister Fiona were at nursery together. Marc and I named our Jake Jake because of her Jake. Are you with me? We go way back.

She's a Leo, a lioness, as her mane of golden curls proves. So insightful, so bright, so funny, *such* a drama queen but God, I love her.

A single mum at twenty-one, she's lived many lives. Actor, playwright and now midwife, she's started over several times but I've rarely seen her shining light dimmed.

She really loves me, does Jess. 'My Em' she says when we're together, which isn't often enough. Repeating my name more than is necessary, as if to hammer home whatever passionate point she's making.

As my treatment took its toll she found it hard to hide her tears. 'Em. Em!' she'd say, her blue eyes glistening and her lips wobbling. 'Fucking hell, Em. It's so unfair. You're strong though, Em darling. You can do this. I KNOW you can do this.'

Having moved out of London to Essex, she came to visit for a couple of days to help and as her trip coincided with my fourth cycle of chemotherapy it made sense that she join me at the hospital.

We drove in her car to the clinic in Wimbledon, stopping at a deli on the way to pick up sandwiches and juice. Pulling in on a yellow line, I got out of the car, purse in hand, to get supplies for the hours ahead.

'Get something good, Em!' She called after me, hazard lights flashing. 'You need to eat, darling. Get chicken, Em, get meat – you need protein.'

The ulcers that filled my mouth and covered my tongue made eating an utterly miserable experience. My taste buds had gone into hibernation and everything tasted like the cardboard wrappings from an Ikea flatpack.

'Fuck it, Em, get some cake as well! Gotta have cake, Em, gotta have cake.'

Jess is what you, what anyone, would call a stunner. There's the hair but also the smile, her bright eyes, her curves, her laugh. I used to feel grey, bland and invisible next to Jess. Sometimes I didn't feel confident enough to be around her. But that was years ago. That was when life's dark times meant that the boy I liked didn't like me back. Or the auditions I'd been to had come to nothing. That was when, I realise now, life was actually perfect but I had no idea.

That was when I was Rapunzel in the top of my flat: single, solitary and self-conscious.

She looked particularly hot on this chemo day. She was wearing a tight (really tight) black skirt, a fitted black top that revealed her black bra underneath and funky heels to give her naturally small stature a boost. Earlier that morning there was a whispered confession: 'Em! I've got no bloody knickers on! I forgot to pack clean knickers, Em. Bloody hell, what a nightmare!'

I was dressed in my standard treatment attire of tracksuit bottoms and sweatshirt. Cosy clothes for chemo, cosy clothes for curling up under the hospital blanket on the hospital chair by the window as the nausea kicked in.

I was a regular by now – a few short weeks in and I was one of the gang.

'Morning, Emma! How are you today?' Elaine the staff nurse called from behind a computer as Jess and I walked into the small, plainly decorated ward.

'Hi, Emma!' smiled Ingrid, one of the pharmacists, as she hurried past us and out of the door.

'Morning, Kate!' cried Mad Julie with the Novelty Socks from over her shoulder, busy with a beeping machine and cursing loudly as she prodded at the uncooperative screen to the mild terror of the elderly gentleman attached to the clearly defunct piece of kit.

'Morning,' I mumbled to them all and slightly nervously at Mad Julie, never brave enough to tell her that I was, in fact, called Emma.

'You look like a Kate!' she'd said once upon realising her mistake. 'Sorry, Emma. I left my bloody brain at home with the cats.'

I laughed it off, reassuring her it didn't matter.

Five minutes later I was Kate once more and remained so for ever after.

Jess was great company at the start of this particular day. Convoluted stories were told, interrupted every time my designated nurse came over to do the standard observations in preparation for the start of chemo. Height, weight, blood pressure, temperature and then – deep breath – 'We'll just pop your canular in, Emma and then we can get going. Is that OK?'

Fucking canulars. I remain, to this day, traumatised by the things. Dig, dig, dig, over and over again and still the damned thing won't work. Why don't they work? Within a few short cycles of chemotherapy our veins do their very best to repel these small but deadly daggers of doom. CANULAR. It's a word I loathe but not as much as the words in the following sentence: 'Sorry, Emma, it's not bleeding back.'

And the nurse would try again. Sometimes she'd get a colleague over to help. Dig, dig, dig. I don't sweat easily but beads of the stuff would appear on my forehead, my heart pounding. Eyes closed, head down, jaw clenched. What am I doing here? What the hell am I doing here?

The tears would often come but only once it was finally in. Relief and rage all mixed up. Childish, blubbery tears of self-pity and upset. Take it out, take the horrible thing out. I don't want it.

This day, with Jessie by my side, was the worst of the digging days. It just wouldn't go in. We were seated in the corner by the window and after twenty minutes or so quite a crowd had gathered. Two, three, then four nurses all peering over, offering their two-pennies' worth as to why it wasn't happening. I didn't notice that Jess had gone a bit quiet. In amongst all of the canular kerfuffle I hadn't noticed that she'd turned a whiter shade of pale.

'You OK, Jess?' I asked as she'd already begun sliding off the plastic visitor's chair and onto the floor in one perfect, gliding movement.

Out cold. My chemo buddy was out cold. Eyes closed and mouth open. It had all been too much for the girl with no knickers on who'd come to keep me entertained and uplifted. She did it in the most memorable and unexpected way.

Light relief. She's always been so good at that. In the darkest of times and in the lowest of moods Jess can always throw sunshine on a situation.

Later, with Jess back upright in her chair, sweet tea in hand and rueful chuckles all round, my left hand took a stabbing one more time. Bingo.

'There we go,' said the nurse, almost as relieved as me. 'It's in, Emma. See? Any pain there? Can you feel anything?'

'No, no pain. Thank you. That feels fine.'

Sometimes distraction is all we need from a dark, painful moment. My Jessie-Bombessie did just that.

chapter twenty
magic all around

'You need an au pair,' said everyone, all the time. Over and over again.

Good plan. I'll just chuck out the Henry Hoover and the ironing board and turn the cupboard under the stairs into another bedroom.

'Can't Jake share a room with the triplets?'

Hmmm. Maybe if he doesn't mind sleeping standing up.

'Can't you rent a bigger house, with an extra bedroom? That way you could have full-time, round-the-clock help?'

Er, not really. I'm financially crippled as it is. Nice thought though.

On and on it went. The childcare issue. Another huge problem for which there seemed to be no easy answer.

'How are you going to manage on the days after chemo when you're feeling horrendous?'

No idea.

'How are you going to get Jake to school?'

God knows.

'How are you going to get up in the night for the babies? You need someone with you, Emma. You need an au pair. Or a maternity nurse. No, hang on – you need a NORLAND NANNY!'

Oh, how I laughed.

After diagnosis and during the first couple of months at the new house it seemed like I had no options that didn't involve the incredible generosity of those closest to me. I had no funds, no savings to draw on, no money of my own to throw at the mess – and what a mess it was.

So really it was quite fortunate that something was going on behind the scenes. The universe was doing that 'thang' again of drawing all the right people together at exactly the right time. Sliding doors. Synchronicity. Whatever you want to call it, miracles were popping up everywhere.

Thea called, an old school friend and colleague at work.

'Hey lovely, have you got a moment? I was round at a friend's house yesterday and happened to be telling her about you and the triplets and Jake. She's just had a baby and just couldn't believe it when I told her what you were going through.'

I held the phone to my ear on my shoulder and carried on rinsing out the dozen or so half-empty baby bottles that were piled up in the sink as Thea talked. I tried to concentrate on what she was saying and block out the grizzles and squawks that were coming from the babies, who were lying on their play mat in the living room. As I listened I found myself visualising her and her pal sitting over coffee in what I imagined to be a beautiful, spacious kitchen. Bright, mid-morning sunlight streaming in through the windows, new baby on the boob. The house neat and tidy, her husband at work. Sore nipples and sleepless nights and maybe a mild case of the baby blues but, most of all, normality. How I longed for normality.

'Anyway, she's got a maternity nurse at the moment, a lady called Sheila. Sheila was there yesterday, overheard us talking and she wants to help you. Do you mind if I give her your details?'

The Lady Called Sheila got in touch and her plan was simple but breathtaking. She wanted to offer her services, free of charge, for the week in October when I was due to be in hospital having the mastectomy and reconstructive surgery. The surgery was scheduled for a few weeks after the chemotherapy was finished. The shrunken tumour/tumours would hopefully be much easier to remove and therefore the results were likely to be more positive. She would come and stay at the house for seven nights and completely take care of the babies until morning when others would step in.

That was the biggest tick ever on another of my lists. The *what the hell am I going to do about the kids when I go into hospital to get my cancerous breast chopped off?* list.

It was a huge weight off my mind. No more thoughts at four in the morning of the babies and Jake being taken into foster care and never seen again. No more imaginings of them being whisked off to France, never to return.

Meanwhile, childcare miracle number two was heading my way. Katy called.

'Camilla's got an offer of help for you and it might solve a lot of your problems.'

Camilla and her husband had always had an au pair for their kids. Their house was huge, their incomes comfortable and so why the hell wouldn't they?

This was their plan and it was off the scale.

A lady called Connie was temporarily staying with them, having just arrived in the UK from Mexico. She was looking for work with a family but needed accommodation too.

'Camilla and Robert don't need Connie's help but they're happy to let her live with them rent-free and she can work for you as a live-out au pair.'

A live-out au pair! Does such a person even exist?

'Really? Are they sure?' Camilla and Robert were Katy's friends; I only knew them vaguely. It seemed like too generous an offer.

'Of course. They want to help; it's perfect. Let me know what you think and I'll —'

'When can she start? No, really. When can she start?'

Connie might as well have floated down from the heavens. A celestial being. Serene, centred, softly spoken and with a heart that was open and ready to give without condition. She arrived and that was it, she fell in love with the babies and they fell in love with her. I exhaled. Everyone did. Connie was here. Miracle number two. Tick.

The miracle momentum gathered. They were pouring in thick and fast and I was at a point when I just went with everything. You want to do my laundry? It's all yours. You want to take the babies for a walk on Sunday morning? Just tell me what time and they'll be ready – in fact I'll be standing by the front door tap, tap, a-tap tapping my toes waiting for your arrival.

You're Natasha Kaplinsky and are due at the TV studios at 5 p.m. but want to come round on your way and start chopping up onions and garlic and rummage through my tupperware drawer looking for matching lids? Be my bloody guest.

Seeing the Channel 5 news anchor batch-cooking bolognese for the freezer with our mutual friend Lucy was a sight I'll always remember. One of the many 'what the hell has happened to my life this is all bonkers' moments that had become the norm.

'I've told Natasha all about you and she's desperate to help,' said Lucy who I'd met at the IVF clinic the year before. Rafa, her beautiful flaxen-haired boy and Ella, Louis and Theo were born, unexpectedly, on the same day and have been known ever since as The Quads. It was a joyous, bonding connection. Another one in the charmed, blessed area of my life that came under the heading of 'friends'.

Lucy lives in Portugal and on her rare visits back to the UK she embarks on a whirlwind tour of family visits, work and the briefest of catch-ups with a few select friends. She very sensibly decided to kill two birds with one stone by inviting 'Tash' along for a catch up with me.

'She really wants to meet you,' said Lucy as we FaceTimed a few days before she flew over. 'She wants to help. Do you mind if I bring her with me? Oh my darling girl, I cannot wait to give you the biggest of squeezes.'

In they swept, both looking gorgeous. Lucy, because she simply is – all smiles and warmth and Natasha because as well as being a natural looker she also had that 'look'. The telly look. Perfect make up, glossy hair and skin – I couldn't take my eyes off her skin. The dewy glow! How do they do that?

I think it's fair to say I wasn't looking my best. Bald as a coot and my skin a rather unappealing shade of yellow. It was mid afternoon and the babies were scattered about and...

(Hang on. Do you mind if we just stop the pretence? I don't have the tiniest clue what the babies were doing on this particular afternoon. How on earth can I remember whether they were asleep or awake or grizzling or cooing or whether Ella was doing that screeching thing she did or whether Theo was trying to roll off their play mat or if Louis was grizzling and fretting or giggling so hard that he fell back and bumped his head. I don't remember! It's a complete and utter blur. But you don't mind that, do you? Surely it's better for me to be honest about the fact that so, so much of that time is a haze to me now. Is that just because time has passed and it's completely normal that the finer details of day-to-day life have been forgotten or is it like a kind of mental shut down?)

What I DO remember is Lucy and Tash arriving and completely taking over. They'd brought mounds of mince, jars of pasta sauce, onions, mushrooms, peppers, garlic and they set to work. Lucy worked like a demon, chopping, dicing, slicing and stirring, calling out every so often from the stiflingly hot kitchen, the key that opened the two tiny windows nowhere to be found –

'Em, where are your chopping boards?

'Em, I forgot tomato puree, do you have any?

'Em, darling! Sorry to interrupt but just checking, have you got enough room in the freezer for three large containers?'

'Right,' said Natasha, my new buddy, as we sat in the living room and she stared at me earnestly. 'What do you need? What can I do? Washing? How about I take your washing away today and I'll drop it back tomorrow morning.'

'No, no, no it's fine, really, no you can't –'

'Don't be silly. It's simply not a problem. Let's strip the beds and change the sheets. Come on, let's do it now.'

And I surrendered, because that's what I'd become so good at.

We went upstairs and I apologised for the mess and she shushed me while I rummaged through the airing cupboard, feeling slightly self-conscious, looking for clean cot sheets and duvet covers and, together, we stripped and then made all the beds and all the cots and that felt nice. Really nice, because who doesn't love clean sheets?

Thea called again.

'We want to do a cake bake for you, at work. Everyone's on board. Is that OK? We'll raise as much cash as we can for you and the babies.'

For so long I'd felt pretty invisible at work, which was completely my own issue as the company was amazing and everyone there absolutely lovely. I was the part-time receptionist with no clear direction. I felt my mark on the company was pretty insignificant. But, clearly, I was considered to be very much a part of the 'family' whether I realised it or not because oh, how they baked. Cakes, buns, muffins, cheesecakes, biscuits, fruit loafs. A couple of weeks after her phone call, Thea sent me a picture of a trestle table up in the Green Room on the fourth floor which was almost buckling under the weight of freshly made delights. The picture was attached to a brief email that read:

We've raised £1,000 in cash for you. I hope it helps. Everyone here sends their love.

Hope it – Sorry, did you say *hope it helps?*

Let me tell you how much it will help, Thea. Let me tell all of you. It will pay for nappies and formula and some new babygros and it will pay for more hours of Connie's wonderful, vital help and it will pay for sleep for me. The thing I crave most. Beautiful, perfect, unbroken sleep.

Yet again, what could I do other than send back a woefully inadequate email? The same blurb as always.

Blah, blah, blah, I'm speechless.

Blah, blah, blah, I don't know what to say.

Blah, blah, blah, I can't thank you enough.

And then I'd slip in some mildly humorous, self-deprecating line about rocking the bald look and who needs eyelashes anyway. That kind of thing.

So I had Connie now and my amazing colleagues had baked lots and lots of cakes. Connie, cakes and chemo. Oh, and lots of bolognese in the freezer. We were getting through. Slowly but surely. We were getting through.

chapter twenty-one
drowning, definitely not waving

Once upon a time the postman knocked and I bounded down the stairs to answer the door.

The End.

No, really. That's it.

After months of laboured breathing, chronic fatigue, of struggling to shuffle from room to room and of a feeling of physical weakness that I thought would never shift... let me tell you, it was quite a moment.

Hang on –

Did I just –

Did I just take the stairs two at a time?

It was leaving my system. I could feel the chemotherapy slowing departing, packing its bags, clearing off out and taking all its nastiness with it. Hooray! Bring out the party poppers to mark the end of active treatment so brutal that not everyone survives it! Bring out a Colin the Caterpillar cake and raise a glass of something sparkly! It's over and done with and life can start again – right away!

Sadly, it wasn't as straightforward as that.

Life doesn't just begin again. A new life starts but it's not a film and it certainly doesn't come with a Marc Curtis script. It's not a feelgood Boxing Day flick with a happily-ever-after ending and bucket lists ripped up because they're no longer needed. It's a fragile, mundane, slow, absolutely terrifying new life that you wouldn't wish on your worst enemy.

'You'll have a bit of a wobble when all this is finished,' Professor Powles told me as I embarked on the last few sessions of radiotherapy while still recovering from the mastectomy. *A bit of a wobble? A bit of a bloody wobble?* I loved that man for saving my life, for his heart-melting bedside manner and unfailing sensitivity but I could think of more candid ways to describe the gut-wrenching anxiety that consumed and exhausted me as I did my best to believe that I really was well and that the cancer had gone.

The mastectomy (slash reconstruction) had been brutal, barbaric even. Best not to think about it too deeply. Nine hours of surgery. Right boob gone. All twenty-six lymph nodes from under my right arm gone. Cancer gone? Apparently so. I can barely remember anything about it now. I remember coming round from the op and being mortified that my trusty lilac cap hadn't been plonked back on my head. Such vanity! I remember Dad, Ro and Fiona's faces smiling down at me. No Jake, though. No babies. I couldn't let them see me like this. Not with the surgical drains collecting a murky yellow and then pink-coloured fluid from the incision sites. Not with the catheter drainage bag hanging from the side of the bed. Not with the bandages around my chest and the wincing expression on my pale, pinched face.

I don't remember any feelings about losing a breast back then. Just get the thing off, get rid, cut it all out, do what you have to bloody do. In fact I wish they'd taken the other one off while they were there. I wish I'd thought to ask, I wish I'd been given that option. It would have felt good to have woken up to both of them gone, both of them replaced with fake, perky, symmetrical 'breasts' that contained no real breast tissue whatsoever. If there's no real breast tissue then surely the risk of recurrence is gone? Ah, what the hell do I know? I don't ask, you see. I never ask.

The recovery was as tough as you might imagine. No lifting for eight weeks. No holding, cuddling or carrying the babies. God, that was hard. Of course I cheated, how could I not? What mum could ignore her babies' outstretched arms day after day, week after week. *I'm strong*, I told myself. *It'll be fine*. And anyway, I just did it when no one was looking.

'We got good clearance,' said Mr Sharma when I shuffled into his office ten days after the op to hear the results of the histology report.

We got good clearance. It sounded like a line from *Top Gun*. 'We're in as good a position as we could be in,' he said, smiling (Mr Sharma not Tom Cruise).

Dad sat there with me, his eyes glistening as we listened. I don't know how I felt really. It was only afterwards that I felt grateful for my ignorance. I had no idea what a histology report was. I didn't realise until much later just how important the results of it were. It was only afterwards, as Dad, Ro and I drove to the village to celebrate with a glass of wine that it hit me. I was… was I… really… cancer-free?

I remember standing on the corner of the street, outside our trusty Café Rouge, leaving Dad and Ro inside while I came out to make a few calls. 'It's gone!' I said to Fiona, Miles, Mel and then, over the course of the next few days, to everyone I knew who was waiting with bated breath. 'Mr Sharma says they got it all and it's gone!'

'We're in as good as position as we could be.' Mr Sharma's words played over and over. I loved that sentence. I loved saying it, repeating it. It doesn't get much better really, does it? I remember the world looking different that day. The colours brighter, the sounds louder. It was one of those technicolour days that life only occasionally gifts – the kind you're lucky if you can count on one hand.

But emotionally, in the months that followed, I felt lost at sea, adrift and completely alone. Being inside my head was not a good place to be. There's no denying the fact that, physically, I was coming back to life. However, the end of my cancer treatment also heralded the start of…

The Wilderness Years.

Thinking back makes me shudder. Ella, Louis and Theo aged one, moving, climbing and falling. And then aged two, three, four… growing and shouting and asking *why, why, why* and yelling *no, no, no.* They had found their voices and their strength too.

Three times a day, three highchairs all in a row — but not close enough to pull out a handful of one another's hair or reach over and scratch a plump cheek with jagged uncut fingernails. One bowl, one spoon and one me. One parent standing, never sitting: no time to sit, so much to do, always so much to do.

Train noises and aeroplanes zooming liquidised vegetables and mushy pasta into one open mouth and then another and then another. Round and round the mulberry bush. Clearing up, mopping up, scrubbing stubborn stains off the grubby carpet with baby wipes and elbow grease.

The boys' hair was dark and curly now, Ella's fair and wavy, while mine had made a comeback, cruelly reminding me that I'd never been a natural blonde. They were desperate to explore, move forward and take on the world while I was trying to find the courage to open the front door, step outside and pick up where I had left off.

'You're looking great, Em! Really well!'

'You've done it, Em! It's over!'

'Wow, aren't you incredible! Look what you've come through!'

No, no, *not* incredible! No, *not* amazing. Scared and lost and angry and frightened and help me please because I don't know what the hell I'm doing. What does it mean or matter that I look OK, that I might always wear lipstick and sometimes even perfume and I smile even when I'm sad and say I'm fine thank you even when I'm not? What do new eyelashes and healing mastectomy scars and fewer hospital appointments matter if I don't know how to find joy in survival or how to let go of the fear?

I don't know how to not be afraid of cancer, of death, of living with uncertainty.

Trying every day, I honestly did try every single day to be a good mum but I always, always felt like I'd failed.

I can still remember so clearly how they felt, those Sunday morning 5.30am wake-ups, all of us down in the living room, curtains closed, still dark outside. Babies, toddlers crawling, my eyes darting, body poised, ready to pounce on a wandering child intent on seeking out danger.

'What are we going to do today, Mummy?'

Oh Jakey.

THAT question.

Deep breath.

'I don't know darling,' I'd say with as much calmness as I could muster, when inside I was screaming: I DON'T KNOW! I DON'T KNOW WHAT WE'RE GOING TO DO TODAY OR TOMORROW OR NEXT WEEK OR NEXT YEAR. I DON'T KNOW ANYTHING ANY MORE. DO YOU HEAR ME, EVERYBODY? I DON'T KNOW!

Who could I talk to early on a Sunday morning? Who could I possibly call at 8.47am when I'd already been up for three hours and the tea had been drunk and the rice cakes and raisins had been doled out and the clock didn't seem to be moving and the forecast was rain, rain, rain and the day stretched selfishly ahead, not caring that every minute felt like an hour and every hour felt like a day.

Who could I call?

Dad, of course.

'Hi Dad, have I woken you?'

'Of course not, my darling' – though sometimes I wasn't sure – 'Did you get much sleep?'

'A bit. Same as always. Up a few times.'

'Poor darling. What are your plans today?'

I could never be irritated with Dad asking me that question. Like I was never irritated by Jake asking me, just overwhelmed by the emptiness of a cruel Sunday.

'No plans, Dad. No plans today.'

'Ro and I will pop down later and have a cup of tea. I'll bring a sweetmeat. What's a good time?'

Anytime, Dad. Now. Come now with Ro and take over and let me hide in a cupboard for ten minutes. Let me walk round the block, stare into space and just have silence. Come now and then come back again later. Pop in and surprise me. Thank you, Dad, for popping in on a Sunday when no one else is around because they're all having cosy family time and pyjama days and snuggles and all I can think is how wrong I must be getting it because a pyjama day has never been an option in our house. How do relaxed, happy, go-with-the-flow pyjamas days happen?

One day. One day we will have our very own pyjama day.

But I did try. Occasionally, I even had moments of intense optimism.

'We're going to bake today, Jake! Cupcakes!'

And we would and it would be carnage but the four of them would love it and then the sugar would kick in and I'd kick myself for adding blue food colouring to the icing as Theo's head started spinning and Ella shrieked repeatedly like a faulty car alarm and Louis fretted and fidgeted and clung on to my legs for dear life.

There would inevitably always be a point on a Sunday afternoon when I would barricade myself in the bedroom and curl up behind the door and they'd bang and scream and cry and kick and yell *Mummy, Mummy, Mummy* from the other side and I'd cry and yell back, *leave me alone, just leave me alone,* feeling like a witch, like a shrivelled old shrew because all I wanted was to be left alone because it was so, so, so hard.

And then finally they'd be in bed and the house would be tidy and the candles would be lit and the chocolate would be out and maybe the wine would be poured and then the guilt would come. Bad mummy. Shouting, screeching and screaming at these poor babies who didn't ask to be born and shouting, screeching and screaming at my beautiful boy Jake who didn't ask for his cosy world of cuddles and kisses and safety and stability and routine to be turned on its head by a mum who got what she wanted and now couldn't cope.

I thought I'd be a much better mum. I honestly thought I was born to be one. From being a teenager and sticking cushions up my jumper to see what I'd look like pregnant, to jabbing my thigh with a giant needle while going through IVF, willing my body to cooperate, I'd always seen motherhood as a goal, a higher purpose in life.

I was convinced I'd be the best kind of bustling, busy, bonnie mum who loved to bake and read stories and draw pictures and play. Play! What's that? I never play. I'm too busy, too tired, too irritable, too distracted, too scared of dying to play.

I thought I would treasure it all so much more.

The fraught moments in Asda, the wet mornings at the playground or the hours spent searching for nits. The relief of being alive and upright and not bald. I thought I'd make scrapbooks of every drawing, of every poem and every *I love you, Mum* note. I thought I would etch each smile on my heart and tattoo each kiss onto my soul.

But it's simply so much harder than I ever imagined. The tiredness steals the joy; it makes the moments of play feel torturous rather than medicinal. The rough and tumble and the shrieks and jostling do just that – they jostle and jar my fractured nerves. And I go to bed, fall into bed and it's not even nine o'clock – sometimes it's half past seven – and I stare into space like a zombie and I wonder if I deserve their love, any of it.

I love you, Mummy, so, so much.
You're the best person in the entire universe.
You're at the top of my heart, Mummy.
Cuddle me, Mummy. Sit with me.

Or simply –

Love you, Mum. From Jake.

And I hate myself because they're all nestled into the top of my heart too and the four of them are the best people in my entire universe and I love them so, so, so, so much. All my soul wants to do is sit and cuddle them for ever and ever but something stops me and I don't know what it is.

Laziness?

Lack of interest?

A stone where my heart should be?

Ice running through my veins instead of blood?

No. No, no, no, no, NO.

This is my theory.

I haven't exhaled. Since they arrived. Since Ella, Louis and Theo arrived and in the months before when everything was falling apart and I couldn't breathe – in all that time, I still haven't exhaled.

Because just as I should have been getting myself on track, just as I should have been pinching myself that my three little miracles were here and alive, just at the very moment when I'd begun to create a feeling of safety in our world, just then – cancer came. It robbed me and it robbed my babies. All four of them. It robbed them of an exhausted but happy mum. Of a mother with space in her brain to find things funny and silly and of a mother who knows that creativity and mess are important. A mother who can see the joy in jumping in muddy puddles and early morning snuggles even though it means dirty clothes or elbowed boobs.

I don't know how to be that mother. I don't know how to play, how to let go and breathe out and allow myself the luxury of truly, madly and deeply connecting with my beautiful, beautiful children.

It's pretty bloody obvious, isn't it?

The more deeply I connect, the more frightening it is to think of leaving them.

So, as tragic as it is, I hold back. I don't even realise I'm doing it.

chapter twenty-two
tapping away the terror

Blog Entry, August 2011, 'All That Glitters…'

SHINE – Cancer Research UK's night-time marathon walk – is drawing near and so today a photographer, along with a lovely lady from the charity's media team, came to the house to take a few publicity snaps of me and the children looking… er… shiny. Ella immediately entered into the spirit of things and within minutes was dressed from head to toe in a silver sequinned skirt and jacket. Louis morphed into a miniature 1970s game show host, donning an oversized silver sequinned blazer and sequinned hat, and Jake wore a silver sequinned waistcoat and a mortified expression (did I mention the silver sequins?). Theo was miserable with a streaming cold, refused to go anywhere near the shiny clothes and seemed to have decided that blowing bubbles out of his nose would be his contribution to raising the profile of what is a fantastic event.

I definitely got the short straw as far as dressing-up fun went. No glittery garments for me. Instead, I was handed a large T-shirt with the SHINE logo and charity name emblazoned on both sides. All well and good and I was proud to wear it but goodness me – is there a less flattering item of clothing to be found than a unisex, oversized T-shirt? If I'd wanted to accentuate my large, wonky boobs and give the impression that I had absolutely no waist then I couldn't have asked for anything better. We did the shoot in the garden and I thought seriously about grabbing a couple of clothes pegs off the washing line in at attempt to create the illusion of a nipped-in midriff. I didn't and silently told my ego to go and hide somewhere.

And so the photoshoot began and all was fine. Jake was being a tad resistant and sulky but a few snarled threats of computer game withdrawal and he soon managed to raise a smile. Louis was scarily enthusiastic about the whole thing and seemed to have found his calling – fluttering his eyelashes, smiling his best showbiz smile and stealing the limelight from the rest of us, hands down.

It all started so well. It fell apart spectacularly. Fifteen minutes in and we had three screaming toddlers and a sullen eight-year-old. I'm not sure that the photographer got one shot with all five of us actually looking at the camera and smiling at the same time. My shiny smile got more strained and tense by the second as I tried to prize a dummy out of Theo's mouth and a stinky, soggy muslin out of Ella's.

'They're not normally like this,' I kept mumbling as the whole shoot crumbled and our sympathetic but slightly startled guests tried to work around the chaos. 'I don't know what's got into them,' I said, laughing nervously as I tried to wrench Louis's jaw from Theo's left shoulder. We ended up having no choice but to barricade the triplets in the living room, Jake in charge, while I sat on a blanket in the garden grinning manically for the camera and doing my best to ignore the three squished faces pressed up against the glass, screaming for me and tearing each other to pieces.

I don't expect to see our faces gracing too many billboards anytime soon. Unless Cancer Research UK decide to turn the whole thing around and plaster pictures of my children at their astonishing worst on every corner – thereby terrifying the public into supporting the amazing work they do. Wait a minute, that could work…

'SINGLE! 4 KIDS! AND NOW I'VE GOT CANCER!!'

Gosh. Thank you *Pick Me Up!* magazine for that low-key, under-stated headline. Much appreciated. Jeez. The article inside was actually lovely and sensitively written but the cover had me giving serious thought to the idea of upping sticks, moving overseas and starting over. Though actually, I think I got off lightly, bearing in my mind that jostling for prime position on the front page along side my stunning tagline was 'I GAVE AWAY MY KIDNEY AT A PARTY!' and 'I BORROWED NATASHA'S WOMB!'

All delightful stuff.

As a result of taking part in the Shine walk for Cancer Research UK and ticking the 'yes' box when I filled in the application form that asked if I'd be happy to share my story, I started doing bits of awareness-raising for the charity, something that I continue to do now, with great pride. I said yes to being interviewed by quite a few of the weekly mags and it felt great to be doing something positive.

Best magazine were one of the first to interview me and, just like the others, it was a mostly uplifting piece, which was what I wanted. I was on the up: treatment had finished and life was back on track. Ish. The running theme was *look at this brave woman, look at how well she's coped!* Not to mention my incredible friends and how they rallied round: *'Emma's Angels!'* And bloody hell, weren't they just.

I've never felt brave about my cancer diagnosis. I simply can't relate to that feeling at all. Bravery doesn't come into it. Petrified, not brave. Does putting one foot in front of the other make you brave? Does having a biopsy or an MRI scan or watching your hair fall out in clumps qualify for some kind of bravery award? I don't think so. I, like so many others, just didn't have a choice and I'm well aware that it was the other jaw-dropping aspects to my 'story' that had people mouthing that flattering but, as far as I'm concerned, undeserving 'B' word.

So when a voicemail came through one grey day in October 2011 I had to listen to it several times to understand what was being said.

It felt like a bit of a joke. A lovely joke but a joke nonetheless.

A bravery award? For me? Uh?

OK, so it wasn't the *Pride of Britain* team calling. I wasn't going to be standing on the stage at Grosvenor House alongside a lollipop lady who'd fought off a masked attacker or a four-year-old who'd given her dad CPR while trapped in a burning building. Carol Vorderman wasn't going to be shimmying across the stage towards David Beckham or Gary Lineker as I waited nervously in the wings. It wasn't that kind of award. But, fuck me! It was an award and, I had to admit, it was really rather exciting.

The Best Magazine Bravest Women Awards 2011. Eleven women chosen to attend a two-day event at a hotel just outside of Croydon. Okay, okay, not Park Lane but who cares? It was the very same hotel where the *X Factor* finalists go for Boot Camp. I was going to follow in the hallowed footsteps of One Direction, Rebecca Ferguson and the legend that was, er, Matt Cardle.

We'd been invited to arrive on a Sunday afternoon in November, meet and mingle with our fellow, ahem, award winners, enjoy a three-course meal and early night followed by photoshoots and interviews the next day, finishing off with the awards ceremony that night hosted by none other than…

Drum roll please…

Mr Eamonn Holmes and his lovely wife… Ruuuuthhhh Lannngggsfoorrddd!

What a scream. How bloody funny.

'So, Emma. Are you available? We would so love you to attend.'

Attend?

Attend?

I'll be there with bloody bells on. Count me in, Helen from the Lifestyle Team at *Best* magazine. Count me bloody in.

Me being me, though, I couldn't just enjoy it. That would have been too easy. Too straightforward. As with most lovely things in my life I seem to need to tarnish the joy with the thick block-brush of anxiety. Slathering the darkest, gloopiest of thoughts all over every potentially happy, uplifting experience and doing my level best to find something, anything, to worry about.

There were two things bugging me in the lead-up to and during the *Best* Awards weekend.

Thing One was anxiety about who else was going to be there. Not social anxiety but the dreaded and actually quite shameful Cancer Comparison anxiety.

What if there was a person there with a gloomier story than mine? What if I met someone who was dying? I was so firmly in the grip of constant thoughts of early death that I felt the need to scan every potential situation, check for danger and prepare myself accordingly. Usually by avoidance.

And Thing Two was my own latest health anxiety obsession, a.k.a. *My Chest Has Been Feeling a Bit Tight Therefore I Must Have Secondary Lung Cancer.*

I'm ashamed to admit this now but my *What If I Meet Someone There Who's Really Ill?* anxiety was so bad that I actually rang the *Best* team a few days before to find out who the other award recipients were. I was clearly not in a good way. What a clumsy phone call.

'Hello, *Best* magazine, how can I help?'

And after the usual pleasantries and unnecessary questions about the itinerary of the weekend I finally got it out.

Cringe Factor? Fair to mortifying.

'Er… sorry, er, this is a really weird question but I get quite worried about my health and stuff and so… er… I just wondered if there were going to be any other women at the awards who have breast cancer?'

Oh, Emma. Really? Did you have to?

Whichever lovely lady I spoke to was totally sensitive and discreet though I hate to think what she was thinking or mouthing to her colleagues.

'Don't worry, Emma, that's fine – let me see, yes, we've got one other lady who's had treatment but she's doing really well at the moment.'

I don't know if making that call helped me in anyway whatsoever. I'm not sure what I wanted to achieve. It was clearly some kind of post-traumatic stress disorder/control-freak response which I know was understandable but that didn't make it any less bonkers.

Mel was my plus-one and thank God for that because I needed her and, as always, she was there. My Mel-shaped rock.

We arrived at the hotel late afternoon on the Sunday and nervously mingled in the foyer as the other er... brave ladies arrived. They all seemed lovely and we made small talk for a couple of hours and shared our reasons for being crowned Courageous.

Back up in our room, with a couple of hours to spare before dinner, I wobbled. Anxiety had taken hold. Sitting on the edge of my bed I started babbling.

'My chest isn't right, it doesn't feel right, it's tight, I can't get a full breath, do you ever get that? What could it be, do you think it's my lungs? What if it's my lungs? It is my lungs, I know it. I've just got a feeling, I know it, I –'

'Darling. Stop.' said Mel. 'Take a deep breath.'

I took a comedy-style breath. Except I wasn't laughing. I was convinced something was wrong.

'Why don't we do some tapping, darling? It might help. Come on, I'll do it with you.'

So we sat on the edge of our beds, facing each other, and I followed Mel's lead as we attempted to tap my fears away. I repeated after her:

'Even though I'm really worried about my chest...'

'Even though I'm really worried about my chest...'

Tap, tap, tap, tap, tap.

'And I'm scared that it's lung cancer...'

'And I'm scared that it's lung cancer...'

Tap, tap, tap, tap, tap, tap.

'I completely and deeply love and accept myself.'

'I completely and deeply love and accept myself.'

Frantic tapping, tappity, tap, tap, tap.

EFT. Emotional Freedom Technique. Tapping with your fingers on different points around your upper body to release emotional blockages. Kind of comical. I imagined my ten fellow award winners, all snugly wrapped in their hotel bathrobes or lying in the bath, while I sat on the edge of the bed trying to tap away the fear.

Mel was always trying to help me manage my anxiety, often

gently suggesting ways that I could manage the thoughts that so often gripped me.

Sounds crazy, but it kind of worked. Or maybe it was the download of Louise Hay's *Power Thoughts* that Mel played as we started to get ready for our meal with the fellow award winners. The 101 positive affirmations that played softly on repeat in the background, reminding me that all was well in my world and that everything was unfolding perfectly.

That's good then. Make-up beautifully applied by Mel, we were ready to go downstairs and mingle with the other guests. I felt a little better.

chapter twenty-three
lovely bernie

At the pre-awards drinks gathering I worked the room. I sashayed and shimmied and charmed and dazzled, sipping on champagne and politely declining the canapés. I mingled with the *Loose Women* ladies and footballers' ex-wives and chatted single parenting with a daytime chat-show host. Honestly, you would have been impressed – I was on *fire*, baby!

Er, except I didn't. And I really wasn't.

There was a lovely buzz in the air, we 'award winners' had all our hair and make-up done, we'd been given pretty frocks to wear and the conversation was flowing. But I was feeling nervous, edgy, and I was struggling to be in the moment and fully enjoy this special night.

And then I spotted her.

From my reaction you might have thought that Madonna had just walked into the room. Or my deceased grandmother, puffing on a Super Kings and wearing one of those funny turban-style hats she used to get out of the back of the wardrobe for trips to town and the like.

There she was.

Bernie.

Bernie bloody Nolan.

Of course, it shouldn't have been a big surprise. I'd already spotted Coleen in a black, sequinned blazer over in the far corner.

I felt myself start to wobble and grabbed Mel's arm, squeezing it tight.

'Look!' I whispered frantically. 'It's Bernie Nolan! Over there, look!'

Mel knew about my Bernie fixation. All those closest to me did. Bernie Nolan was my barometer of wellness and likely survival. If Bernie was OK then I was too. Look, look at her lovely blonde hair tied back into an impressive chignon! Look at her healthy complexion and clear eyes! She looked as well as well could look and that was bloody marvellous. Cheers all round. I probably should have raised my glass to her from my side of the room and turned back to my conversation about brain injuries with Beverley Turner. But I couldn't. I needed to speak to her. I needed to meet Bernie and make a connection.

'I need to talk her,' I muttered to Mel out of the corner of my mouth while keeping my eyes firmly fixed on poor Bernie. 'Can you ask one of the *Best* team to introduce us?'

I didn't mean to treat Mel like my newly employed personal assistant – I think I was just rooted to the spot, frozen.

'Of course, darling,' Mel replied, indulging her slightly unhinged best friend and doing her best not to look at me with pure pity in her eyes.

Mel sorted it out. Bernie and I were introduced. I crumbled like a nine-year-old girl meeting Taylor Swift while Mel looked nervously on and Bernie looked like a rabbit caught in the headlights.

'We *(sob)* were *(splutter)* ill… at… the… same… time. I've *(sob)* been *(sniff)* following your progress and –'

Bernie put her hand on my arm.

'Oh, love. And how are you doing now?'

'I'm OK. I worry that it's going to come back though. All the time. It never stops. Do you?'

'Do *I*?' Bernie almost laughed with recognition. 'Oh, in my mind I've had bone cancer, brain, kidney, lung. The whole bloody lot. I drive myself and my husband mad.'

It was such a relief to hear that I wasn't the only one and that despite the media's constant portrayal of Bernie's positive *cancer can't beat me* message she was still battling her own inner demons. That horrible, spiteful little fucker of a voice telling you that every single twinge, ache or pain is *something*. Something that might mean the beginning of the end.

Bernie gave me a big hug goodbye and, smiling brightly, she said, 'Look at us, we're doing great, don't you think? Keep strong.'

When Bernie was diagnosed with secondary breast cancer the following year I was completely devastated. Sad for this lovely woman with a family and so much life ahead but also, selfishly, devastated for myself. I felt like I'd just been given the same diagnosis. Her cancer was vicious and had reappeared in most of the bodily parts she had jokingly confessed to worrying about.

It can only be a matter of time, I thought, pacing the room and crying down the phone to Fiona late on the same Sunday night that the news appeared online. And the same to Miles the next morning, still obsessing, fixating and googling.

'It's not you, Em. You're not Bernie, darling. It's horrendously sad but this isn't your story.'

But their words fell on deaf ears. I felt like Professor Powles had just knocked on my door, out of hours, and handed me a letter with the date of my death on it.

The awards ceremony itself felt very special and incredibly humbling. It was a mini version of every awards bash you've ever seen. Eleven small round tables, blindingly white tablecloths, napkins, name places and our glasses being topped up with reassuring frequency. Six on each table – a 'Brave Woman', her plus-one, a couple of members of the magazine team and a celeb. The outskirts of Croydon really was the place to be that night.

We had Kristina Rihanoff from *Strictly Come Dancing* on ours which gave us all a little thrill – Mel in particular, megafan that she is. I'd managed to wrangle two extra 'standing-room only' invitations for Fiona and my niece Jasmine so they hovered by the door to start with but then managed to pull up a couple of chairs and squeeze in next to us just as Eamonn and Ruth took their places on the mini stage, microphones in hand. One by one our stories were told and we went up to collect our awards. I hadn't prepared much of a speech. My main focus was on trying not to start crying the minute I opened my mouth, which of course I did. I felt like a bit of a fraud next to the other chosen women. I'd been unlucky, that was all. Some of the other recipients had been hit by the most unimaginable tragedies. We all sat with lumps in our throats as Ruth and Eamonn took turns to introduce us, telling potted versions of everyone's stories while we scrabbled around for tissues.

Kris Hallenga's story was particularly hard to hear.

Aged just twenty-three when she was diagnosed with stage four breast cancer, she and her identical twin Maren founded CoppaFeel! – a charity that focuses on the early detection of breast cancer by encouraging young women to regularly check their breasts, to know what normal feels like for them.

Kris turned her personal tragedy around with incredible focus, dignity and passion, and CoppaFeel! continues to spread the word and boob love by visiting schools, universities and festivals. How bloody amazing.

It turned out that Kris was the young woman I'd been told about when I made the bonkers phone call to the *Best* office the week before. As soon as I saw her I felt ashamed of myself. Embarrassed. Ridiculous even. What exactly was I so afraid of? Why did I feel the need to hide from another human being in such a cowardly way? A woman almost young enough to be my daughter and yet I felt I needed prior warning, protection, so that I could prepare myself for being in the same room as her. Where was my humanity and heart? The only excuse I can give is to be honest about how much of a mess I was in at that time. Consumed by thoughts of what I imagined was going on inside my body. But I knew this whole fingers-in-the-ears approach needed to stop. Was I really going to shrivel into a corner and indulge my own fears to such an extent that it affected how I behaved towards someone I'd never even met? It was a real low point. Once I met Kris, those shrunken, panicked thoughts vanished. Of course they did. She was simply a beautiful, bright young woman who'd had really shitty luck and was not allowing it to defeat or define her. Her courage left me trailing.

Fear was making me self-indulgent. It was all about *my* anxiety, *my* experience, *my* 'what if' mentality. If only I could have just stepped outside of myself that weekend. Extended myself like these other women had, outwards, reaching out to others and making a difference. The fear was crippling me and I was so firmly in its grip that it didn't occur to me not to let it.

chapter twenty-four
my mixed-up mind

Blog Entry, August 2012, 'When We Were Good…'

The long oak coffee table that was the living room centrepiece in my 'old' life is now back with me where it belongs. The cluttered, colourful flat we lived in as a family of three, before the triplets, before the break-up and before that little blip called cancer is being sold and, well, it really does feel like the end of a pretty monumental era. Living in a rented house for the last two years means I haven't really made my mark on the place I now call home. Moving in with the babies and Jake and experiencing the start of what is affectionately known as 'chemo brain', the last thing on my mind was interiors and decor. A few snazzy cushions and some twinkly lights is about as far as I've gone in the style stakes and it shows…

So tonight my beloved table was brought to the house and positioned perfectly by the sofa and TV. I dimmed the lights, placed a big, fat church candle in the middle of it and sat down. An unexpected tidal wave of nostalgia, sentiment and sadness washed over me and it was a little overwhelming. Memories poured in thick and fast and what took me by surprise was that the majority of them were happy ones. It's so much easier just to think of how bad things got. A lot less painful to remember only the terrible times. But there were good times too. Lots of them.

When I was Ella's age, my mum used to read nursery rhymes aloud to me and the one I never tired of hearing was about the little girl with the curl:

There was a little girl,
Who had a little curl,
Right in the middle of her forehead.
When she was good,
She was very good indeed,
But when she was bad she was horrid.

When we were good we were very good indeed, but when we were bad we were
bloody awful.

I'm pleased to have my wooden table back. Now I just need to find a wooden
box to put these mixed-up thoughts in...

Tuesdays and Saturdays. That was the awkward, clumsy and far from ideal routine we seemed to fall into after we separated.

On a Tuesday, Marc would usually come over in the afternoon and stay until bedtime. Kind of. Sort of. So ambiguous, so undefined.

And oh, the tension. Jake's little face, a nervous smile and eyes always darting between Mummy and Papa. How's today's visit going to go? How are these two fools going to cope today? The tightrope of tension stretched from the back of the garden to the end of the close. Would they make it? Would they get through without falling and crashing... again?

Marc would often turn up with a couple of bags of groceries. Nice stuff: fresh bread, cheese, yoghurts for the kids and maybe some chocolate for me. Things I couldn't afford to buy very often. He knew what I liked. I appreciated it, relied on it even. He'd offer to cook, help with bedtime and would pour me a glass of wine at seven o'clock.

Was it too little too late? I was certainly grateful for a selection of goodies that delighted the kids and got my mouth watering but the cheese and olives left a bitter taste when really what I needed was a show of stability and support without conditions. And was it worth the pleasure of a much-needed glass of red wine with dinner – the three of us eating together just like old times – if two hours later things got very tense?

'I can stay the night. Sleep on the sofa. I can help you in the morning.'

'No, it's fine. I'm fine. Thank you.'

The new formal me: minimal eye contact and detached, disengaged.

And then, later on, the silence. Stony silence. Babies asleep, Jake drifting off. No distractions, no interruptions. Bugger. Where were the interruptions when you needed them?

'You don't want to talk?' he'd always ask.

And I didn't. I really and truly didn't. I couldn't talk any more. There was nothing to say that hadn't been said over and over again. It was beyond exhausting. It was simply too late.

'Why, Emma, why won't you talk?'

And I'd feel my anxiety levels start to rise because he showed no sign of going and it was half past eight or ten past nine or quarter to ten and everything was quiet upstairs and these were my precious moments of recovery from the day and I needed them desperately and I didn't have the tiniest fragment of spare energy to talk to the man I'd spent years begging to talk to me. Oh, the irony.

'I'm tired, Marc,' I'd say, standing up, hoping he'd follow my lead. 'I really need to go to bed. We'll see you at the weekend, OK?'

But he wasn't a fool, far from it, and he knew what I was doing and he knew too well that I just wanted him to go. I needed him to go without being asked. To kiss his kids goodnight and make them feel safe and loved and then go. But he couldn't. Well, he could but he wouldn't, and I know he was clinging on for dear life but I couldn't save him or tell him it was all going to be all right because it wasn't. Not between us. Not ever again because we were broken, still broken. We'd been broken for ages and we weren't going to be unbroken ever again.

I had endless conversations with anyone who'd listen, hours of therapy that was supposed to support my emotional recovery from cancer but which instead turned into a weekly analysis of my emotions and our relationship. 'I'm confused,' I'd sometimes say.

'I feel so guilty,' I'd always say.

'Why guilty?' I'd be asked.

Because it hadn't always been bad between us. Because there was lots that was really and truly lovely. And most of all because we now shared four children and being apart had never been the plan.

Vocalising my confusion would always lead to it being gently suggested to me that I write a list of the pros and cons of us staying together. A list, for God's sake? I was in complete and utter turmoil and a list of pros and cons was supposed to provide me with clarity, as though it were as simple as deciding which brand of baby formula to switch to?

Well, I must have written a hundred lists.

I was desperate. Desperate to break free of the cycle we were in and desperate to feel some kind of relief and peace.

My lists, scribbled on the back of an envelope or till receipt from Lidl, were always more or less the same and usually started with the Pros:

He's their dad and we should all be together.

Sometimes things feel really good between us.

And the absolute killer –

I spent so long trying to convince him to try for another baby – I OWE it to him to keep trying.

I spent years feeling agonisingly confused. Or at least that's what I thought the gut-wrenching feeling was. Now, in retrospect, I realise that the emotion wasn't confusion but guilt. I knew what needed to happen. I knew that we couldn't be together but the guilt was so monumental – heart versus head/head versus heart – that it crippled me.

Marc would arrive on a Saturday morning and sometimes it was lovely. There were many times when I didn't understand why we weren't together. Three or four weeks would go by with minimal upset and I'd find myself wondering what the hell was wrong with me, why wasn't I taking him back? Surely life would be easier on so many levels if I just took him back?

My heart would lurch when I saw him rolling around on the floor with the boys or giving Ella a giant kiss, ruffling Jake's hair and calling him 'my boy'. He was their dad, their Papa; he belonged with them. He'd arrive at the house, fresh-faced after as much sleep as he needed, a leisurely bath and the weekend papers. Maybe an omelette with his coffee. Civilised, stress-free.

And I'd find myself struggling to articulate the reasons why I couldn't give 'us' another go.

Couldn't or wouldn't?

Couldn't.

Definitely couldn't.

'I can't go back,' I'd say again and again. Sometimes angrily, sometimes stubbornly and often as I was weeping with exhaustion while changing a nappy or staring at the clock at midnight wondering when I'd be allowed to end yet another late-night phone call.

'I can't, I can't, I can't go back,' I'd say, repeating it like it was a mantra for survival.

Which it was. My longing for a guarantee of health and yes, therefore 'survival', was so great that walking back, voluntarily, into a status quo that I *knew* with every fibre of my being couldn't ever evolve into something truly healthy would be an act of madness.

When we were getting on well I felt wretched. The bad times faded away, I could barely remember them and instead I felt like a two-headed monster, denying the man I'd once loved so much the simple joy of waking up under the same roof as his children.

'Take me back, Emma. I miss my children.'

'I'm sorry, I'm sorry, no, it won't work.'

It felt like my punishment. More so than cancer did. My punishment for wanting a baby. You got what you wanted so now you've got to put up with this stuck, toxic situation for ever. You're tied together. Intrinsically linked for evermore.

How dare you reject this man who went along with your desires? This is your penance and there's nothing you can do about it.

It felt as though there was simply no escape.

We used to have a giant collage of photos hanging on the landing in the flat. This was before the days of Instagram when actual pictures were an actual 'thing' and compiling albums and choosing picture frames was a hugely satisfying task. For me anyway. I spent hours making it and it was filled with snapshots of our life as a family – one happy, laughing shot after another, haphazardly but carefully arranged to show the three of us at our filtered best.

I'd struggle to look at the collage now. It's in storage somewhere at Dad's. I've asked Jake if he'd like to have it hanging up in his room but he said no. Would it be too painful for him to have a daily reminder of his life before? Or is that me, once again, projecting my stuff onto his adolescent – *why the hell would I want embarrassing baby pictures in my bedroom* – head?

We look happy in those photos. I look happy. We weren't good or bad. We were good and bad. In some ways a great match and in other ways like oil and water.

But whatever way you looked at it, we were stuck. It was a stale-mate, a stagnant situation that was slowly but surely draining the life out of both of us and it was inevitable that, one day, the dam would burst.

chapter twenty-five
singing for my soul

Blog Entry, November 2012, 'Sing When You're Winning...'

Just as well I go to choir once a week, as I seem to be prohibited from opening my mouth to warble a tune at home, while strolling in the park, driving my car or anywhere else within earshot of my fabulous four. I feel a little crushed but kind of get it. I remember being seven or eight and absolutely mortified as my mother rehearsed her lines for her starring role in the Broadway Theatre Company's latest, er – 'hit' production. Just to be clear, that was the Fulham-based amateur dramatics Broadway Theatre Company and not some cool, Critics' Choice ensemble based in New York, New York. How I used to cringe as she belted out showstopping tunes from The Pyjama Game, Bye Bye Birdie *and* Guys and Dolls *while making the tea or whipping up a Victoria sponge.*

And now here I am, a generation on, kidding myself that I'm still rather hip when in fact even my two-soon-to-be-three-year-olds are mortified by hearing me belt out the upper alto version of one of Adele's biggest hits or a classic from the Bee Gees.

I'm used to it with Jake. He cuts to the chase, no pussy-footing around, and simply tells me in no uncertain terms to SHUT UP. Missy Ella fixes me with a steely glare and shushes me at top volume, finger firmly on lips, other hand on hip. Theo says nothing but places his grubby little hands over my mouth while shaking his head and Louis (sensitive, troubled soul that he is) looks terribly concerned and in a pleading, heartfelt kind of way says, 'No singing, Mumma – no my not like it.'

OK, kiddiwinks – I get the message. I'll keep quiet. The last thing I want to do is provide you with a million memories of mortification. Little buggers.

A little tip for the four of you though. Please take note – Mummy singing equals mummy in a decent mood. Think about it, kiddos. That's all I'm saying.

'Mr Blue Sky' saved my life.

OK, I might be over-egging it slightly there but I think it's fair to say that my Wednesday nights spent as a member of the Wimbledon branch of Rock Choir came pretty close to saving my sanity.

I'd always wanted to join a choir. Always loved singing – from being teeny tiny and knowing all the words to every 1950's musical ever written courtesy of Mum's love of show tunes to dreaming of being Pepsi or Shirley and go-go-ing behind George and Andrew on *Top of the Pops* on a Thursday night at the peak of my obsession with Wham! For a child, then teenager, so shy and averse to being the centre of attention, I had surprisingly flamboyant dreams.

Mum and Dad didn't bat an eyelid when I said I was going to leave school at sixteen. Partly because when it came to mine and Fiona's education they weren't exactly tiger parents but also because they'd both followed their own creative paths – albeit with very different degrees of success – and they probably just assumed we'd find our way too. Hmmm. In hindsight, they probably should have frogmarched us both into further education with no bloody say in the matter.

Mum was twenty-one when she arrived in the UK from New Zealand having been awarded a bursary to study at the Guildhall School of Music and Drama. She'd already worked a lot in theatre and radio back home and had big plans for a theatrical career in the UK. Once Fiona came along, those dreams took a back seat and that was pretty much the end of what seemed like a promising career.

Dad, on the other hand, won a scholarship to art school in the north-east at fourteen, spent his national service with the Royal

Marines and then slowly but steadily found himself designing sets in repertory theatre, working at the now defunct ABC Television followed by several years at the Royal Court Theatre in Chelsea. He bought a disused church hall in Hammersmith when Fiona was tiny, turned it into his studio and for the next forty years it was his creative playground, his paradise. There probably wasn't a theatre in the West End that Dad hadn't painted a set for. His work was stunning, breathtaking and his talent off the scale. He worked incredibly hard, solidly and consistently, and quickly built up a reputation of being the best scenic artist around. He made it all look so easy. And really, without in any way diminishing his ability, it was easy to him. He's an artist and it was, without question, what he was born to do.

How wonderful it must be to spend your working life doing something so incredibly well and for as long as you want to do it. To know that you've followed your dream and are on the path you were born to be on. Obvious, tangible, no-holds-barred talent makes my jaw drop but if dreams are all that's driving you then reality can be a cruel mistress.

I had the dreams but the real, discernible talent was lacking, certainly when it came to vocals.

Had *The X Factor* been around in my latter teenage years, I would have been one of those pitifully deluded auditionees that is genuinely stunned when Simon and co break the news that they are, in fact, shite at singing. Sure, I could sing in tune and hold the odd note but a career in music was never going to be on the cards. Or on the stage for that matter. Talent is part of it but confidence is also required and I simply didn't have what it took.

So history really was repeating itself when, like Mum and her am-dram Thursday nights in Fulham, I began 'expressing myself' once a week in an amateur choir.

But the fact is, I was in heaven. Really. Rock Choir was my 'step one' back out into the world. It was my time to practise being me again. I could start over. Connect with people who didn't know all that had gone on and who took me at face value without flickers of concern etched on their faces. People who had their own woes and struggles but were, like me, just thrilled to spend two hours a week singing every cheesy middle-of-the-road classic known to man.

Ella, Louis and Theo were still toddlers when I turned up alone for a free taster session. Hair still tellingly short, I was nervous and unsure but possessed just the tiniest nugget of 'fuck it' attitude needed to get me through the church door.

I seemed to find a new gang pretty much straight away. Linda, Helen, Michelle, Sharon, Zoe and Christine – a group of lovely ladies I'm not sure I would have crossed paths with had we not shared a mutual love of singing. We'd sit, every week, in the front row of our vocal section, saving seats for one another and whispering catch-up gossip between songs and miming 'are you going to the pub after?' as we leant forward and hid our faces behind our song sheets. Under the leadership of our absurdly talented choir leader Jim, we'd sing with gusto and close our eyes and feel alive and in the moment and I honestly think for each and every one of us there, choir was a piece of magic in our lives. A chance to exhale and just sing our bruised little hearts out. Maybe I'm projecting, maybe the hearts thumping to the Radio Two rhythms weren't all bruised but I'm pretty sure that everyone there had a reason to leave their cares at the door and take a pew.

Then afterwards, we'd hit the pub. The pub! Suddenly, I found myself with a social life and it was a joy. New friends, new conversations, a new me. I felt alive at choir, glowing and radiant. I felt strong, clear and focused and I knew what I wanted for myself and for the babies and Jake and as I absorbed the harmonies to 'Build Me Up Buttercup' I knew, really, really clearly what I didn't want. I didn't want cancer and I certainly didn't want drama. I wanted freedom, *emotional* freedom and the chance to shape my life, my kids' lives, into something amazing.

Sue was there too. My buddy Sue. She'd stood on my doorstep one sunny morning and listened as I regaled her with stories of the choir I'd joined and how it was responsible for the spring in my step that was clear for all to see.

'I like the sound of that,' she said, beaming, as she stood outside the house, coffee flask in hand.

'You should come along,' I said. And she did.

Sue wasn't a friend at first. She was a saviour. As the manager of the Wandsworth branch of Home-Start, she swept into my life when the babies were just a few months old and shortly before the C-bomb dropped. Home-Start is the most incredible charity with nearly three hundred branches across the UK supporting local families that are going through a difficult time. We must have ticked so many boxes, the babies and me. Single mum, toxic relationship breakdown, triplets, living in a top-floor flat that was clearly too small – yep, Home-Start can help. Sue arrived with her clipboard and trusty coffee flask and briskly went through the process that would ultimately lead to me being matched with a Home-Start volunteer. She was in her late fifties when we met. She was formidable, bossy and blunt but she did so much. She had a mind and heart so big and an absolute passion for making people's lives better.

Sue led me to something huge later on. Something wonderful and life-changing. I want to thank her every day but I can't because she's gone. Sue isn't here any more. Just like John from over the road and my 'barometer of wellness' Bernie. Just like them, she went far too quickly and far too painfully.

Cancer is a bastard.

Sue made sure that Ella, Louis and Theo had birthday cakes when I was too overwhelmed or sleep-deprived to make them. Home-Start volunteers delivered three separate cakes on the morning of their hastily arranged party. My three had no idea how lucky they were. To them it was normal to each have their own personalised cake. It didn't really matter that on Louis's

Fireman Sam cake there was a number three rather than a five. Or that Ella's *Frozen*-inspired sponge was ever so slightly raw in the middle. It meant that each of them had an 'ooh, aaah' moment. As the lights went down and everybody broke into song, all my little monkeys had something a little special. Their very own cake. Indulgent? Maybe. It was something lovely and for three short years, a tradition that Sue made happen.

She also made sure that they got taken out on day trips provided for the Home-Start families. Off to the farm or zoo, all three of them, backpacks on, walking hand in hand, excited and babbling. My three growing babies.

'Sue has arranged something for you, darlings.'

'Sue with the cats?' asked Ella.

'Yes, angel. Sue with the cats.'

Scary Sue is what we sometimes called her. But it was always said with affection, with love. And a great deal of respect.

So Sue went from Home-Start saviour, bringing me two hours of help a week with a hand-picked volunteer, to fellow amateur singer, to true friend, to… well, more of that later. All I can say is that without Sue, my life right now would look very, very different.

chapter twenty-six
ah, so *this* was
our rock bottom

I don't think either of us wanted to make the other cry. I don't think either of us got any kind of satisfaction at all from what was going on.

The end had to come, of course it did. The *real* end, I mean. It was clear to all from very early on that there was never going to be a neat and tidy resolution to the problem that was Marc and me. We were so far removed from Chris and Gwyneth and their 'conscious uncoupling', it was laughable. Except it wasn't. There was no guffawing, just stress, angst and tension with an enormous, foreboding, capital T.

A new year dawned and, there was no denying it, I had a fire in my belly. I felt a shift, a strengthening, a change. Maybe it was the knowledge that I was entering my fifth year since diagnosis. The magic five! That mythical point that we're led to believe equals immunity from any further brushes with cancer or at the very least puts us back on a level playing field with the truly fit and well. Maybe it was seeing the children move into different stages of their development. The triplets were now aged four and in full-time nursery, Jake was now ten and a half and in his last year of primary school. I mean, really – talk about milestones. I was back at work and writing bits and pieces on the side. I had a regular column in a magazine for parents of multiples, I was blogging as much as I could and still loving every single second of my time with Rock Choir.

Also, after finally selling the flat and with a fair old financial contribution from Dad, I'd managed to buy our house and the kids and I went from being tenants to having the wonderful security of knowing we could stay in our little matchbox home for ever, if that's what we wanted.

Cancer was no longer the first thing I thought of when I woke up in the morning. Cancer was fading into the background and the dreams and ambitions I had for myself and the kids were becoming clearer and more focused by the day.

All of these positives and more were stoking the fire inside me. I was growing in strength and confidence in so many ways and yet I still had a ten-tonne emotional weight strapped to my soul.

So maybe my January 2014, *new year, new me!* steely determination was why the lack of closure between Marc and me felt so intolerable. Four years on. Four years post-separation and still we were tethered and bound. Cliché of clichés but God, life really is too bloody short. I simply couldn't stand the thought of another year of tension, of walking on eggshells, of making each other miserable and of saying yes when I wanted to say no. It felt like a criminal waste of life not to have the freedom to be my true self, of having to stay small, contained and constricted when all I desperately wanted to do was fly.

'We can't go on like this,' I said one afternoon when he and I were alone in the house. I was sorting clean washing into piles in the moments before we were due to leave to collect Ella, Louis, Theo from nursery and then Jake from school.

I didn't want to engage but desperately needed to get it out. To feel the fear and do it anyway. I couldn't go on another minute longer allowing my fear of the repercussions to stop me from speaking out.

I lit the touch paper with that one sentence.

'What do you mean we can't go on like this, Emma? We have four children. What do you expect?'

There was no going back now. *Come on, Em, come on. You can do this. Just say it. Everything you want to say, now's the time. You've got nothing to lose.*

'We need to change the routine. We've been apart for years; it's not healthy. I want you to see the kids regularly but away from here. You can pick them up and take them out for the day, or back to your flat. They'd love that.' My heart was pounding but I continued as I headed upstairs with a pile of clothes, not wanting to stand still and look him in the eye. He followed me upstairs into the bathroom.

'It's not normal for separated couples to function like this,' I said, trying to keep things calm but at the same time speaking my truth. Speaking My Truth was imperative suddenly, as though I'd had an epiphany.

'We both need to move on. I want to move on.'

Oh shit.

I can't really say much more about the events that unfolded on that grim Tuesday afternoon. And that's probably a good thing. I think it's for the best. Of course it is. My intention with this book was never to expose the darker sides of our relationship. Or put our lowest moments under the spotlight for all to see. And Marc is, of course, entitled to privacy and to move on with his life as he chooses. And we have four children. Four brilliant, fantastic, beautiful children for whom life will bring its own challenges, its own bumps in the road. They certainly don't need their silly parents' relationship breakdown put out there for all to see.

All I will say is that by the time the end of that day came and by the time the house was silent and still and as I sat staring into space, going over and over what had happened I kept thinking the same thought.

A thought that that was way, way overdue.

It's over.

It's really over. Finally.

And mixed with that thought there was a feeling of relief. Of gratitude almost. I was grateful to him.

Thank you. For helping me draw a line in the sand.

Enough was finally Enough.

And so how were things left between us? It's really quite simple.

Marc is allowed to see the kids but not allowed to contact me directly. He needs to make arrangements to see Jake, Ella, Louis and Theo via a third party.

I still hope that one day some peace and resolution will come. That one day Jake, Ella, Louis and Theo will sit round a table with their Papa and his family in France and forge their own happy, strong memories. For now, I can't control that or make it happen but I have hope. And I know that they do too.

chapter twenty-seven
gok bloody wan?!

I don't miss a trick.

For someone whose fried chemotherapy brain mostly feels like it's full of melted marshmallows and who no longer has the ability to retain facts, names or any kind of useful information – I still don't miss a flipping trick when it comes to what I can only call *goings on*.

Oh Mel.

Mel, Mel, Mel. My beautiful soul sis. The most honest, straight-forward, simply hasn't-got-it-in-her-to-be-murky-about-anything person I think I've ever met.

Hi darling. Just a quickie – what do you think of those TV makeover shows? Would you ever consider doing one?

I bet she agonised over how to word such a seemingly innocuous text.

I have to say I did a double-take.

Makeover shows? Gok bloody Wan assessing me in my bra and knickers *makeover* shows?! Jeez, I know I've been through the mill and my body ain't what it used to be but really? Cheeky cow.

It was the spring of 2014 and I was at my friend Hannah's house – *with* the kids. She'd invited us all over for lunch and a play. No one ever invites us over for lunch and a play. She lived right over the other side of London. North, north London. We're south. South, south. It took *ages* to get to her place, *ages* to get back and my kids took no time at all to trash her stunning home while her two immaculately behaved boys sat huddled next to each other on the sofa, traumatised by the invasion. But it was so good of her. So kind and a happening so rare and precious that it wasn't the time to get into text 'chat' with Mel, even if I'd wanted to. I sent Mel back an uncharacteristically brief response.

Er, not really. Not my kind of thing x

Do you see what I did there?

One kiss. I replied with just one kiss.

In our shared language, I might as well have not bothered. Not signing off a text with several kisses or at least a heart emoji or two meant only one thing. I had the hump.

Later on, back at home, she called. I was cleaning the loo while Dad and Ro were downstairs keeping an eye on the kids. I couldn't help myself; I was a bit off.

'Hi darling!' She was bright and breezy but I wasn't buying it. She sounded edgy, not like Mel at all.

'So,' she said.

'So,' I replied, squirting green toilet cleaner under the rim and wondering at what point my three boys would learn to aim inside the bowl.

'So. Er... makeover shows. You don't fancy it then?'

Didn't she get the message earlier? I glanced at myself in the bathroom mirror. Do I really look that much of a state?

'No, I bloody don't!' I snapped, my voice leaping up an octave. 'I'd hate to stand in my bra and knickers on telly! It would be my worst nightmare.'

Surely she knew that? Surely Mel, *Mel* – my spiritual sister – knew that I was the last person on earth who would want the spotlight on me in such a way. I was baffled, affronted and mildly pissed off.

There was a split-second pause silence followed by a shriek.

'Not *that* kind of makeover show! Not tits out on the catwalk for fuck's sake! I'm talking about *house* makeovers! The house, *your* house! God, babe... ha ha ha, that's so funny!'

She was tickled. I was relieved but puzzled. Oh. That was different, of course, but what did she mean 'what did I think about makeover shows'? Why was she asking?

'Er, not sure... maybe. Why? What —'

'Look, I just need a yes or a no. That's all. Please don't ask me any questions. Just a yes or no.'

'Er... not sure, maybe... er, I guess so, I —'

That was it.

'Great, fab, that's all I needed to hear! Byeeeee!'

And she'd gone.

I put down the phone and flushed the chain, watching the green foamy bubbles rise and then fall.

Heading back downstairs I couldn't help saying something to Dad and Ro.

'Er... I think Mel might be planning some kind of house makeover for me. She's being really weird.'

I was met with silence and uncharacteristically vacant expressions from both of them and for once my antennae failed me. As I started tidying up Theo's toy trains, Louis's collection of elephants and retrieving Ella's stinky cloth from under the sofa it didn't occur to me in a million years that they might know all about it and that behind the scenes all sorts of shenanigans were already occurring.

Further down the line, as the pieces began to fit together, I found out that Dad was worried, Fiona too.

'It's too intrusive!' said Dad.

'What about the neighbours?' said Ro.

'God, it would be my worst nightmare,' said Fiona, shuddering at the thought of a camera crew rummaging through her drawers – the wooden kind, of course.

'You need to find out if Emma wants it done,' they told Mel. 'Otherwise it could be a disaster.'

'But it's supposed to be a surprise,' said Mel. 'It'll ruin the surprise.'

To tell or not to tell wasn't the only tricky aspect of the impending house transformation.

ITV had responded pretty much straight away to Mel's application to *60 Minute Makeover*. They were keen to go ahead and thought the kids and I would make ideal recipients but time was of the essence and it needed to be action stations from the get-go.

'Right, Mel. We need you to be at Emma's house on Thursday when she's at work. Helen, our producer, will meet you there and you can tell us more about Emma and the kids, her style and what changes you think the house could benefit from most.'

Oh. Oh bugger.

'Er... but I live in Yorkshire,' answered Mel. 'Not sure I can make it down for Thursday.'

Poor Mel. She had no idea it was all going to get so flipping complicated. She had just tried to do something lovely and now it looked like it could all fall apart at the first hurdle.

She began frantically getting in touch with the handful of my friends she knew or had numbers for.

'Would you be happy to be the "friend" featured on the makeover? You'd need to be there on the day of filming and help the production team in the build-up to the big day? It'd have to be a secret, of course. Em can't know anything. Let me know as soon as you can.'

One by one my wonderful but camera-shy buddies politely declined her request for them to step into her shoes as my 'special friend' and be filmed for the makeover. The 217 miles between Wandsworth and North Yorkshire were proving to be a rather enormous stumbling block and came close to scuppering the whole thing. Mel was running out of options.

Until she remembered one special person who just might be willing to jump on board. It was a long shot, but definitely worth a go.

chapter twenty-eight
super sue to the rescue

Sue said yes. Of course she did. And actually, I can't think of anyone better qualified to have taken over the reins.

Who better to supervise and plan a top-secret event? Which better no-nonsense 'let's just get on with it, what's next on the list' and 'yes, I'll have a coffee but only if it's not that instant rubbish' kind of person to make things happen?

Sue stepped into the breach and just like that it was all systems go – *60 Minute Makeover* a go-go in fact.

Meanwhile, I was doing okay. Busy, busy, busy but okay, and – apart from managing the ongoing and very tedious *am I going to die very soon from a brief but brutal cancer recurrence?* shizzle that played on a continuous loop in my head – I was actually in a pretty good place.

So picture this. It's bright and early on a Thursday morning. It's quarter to eight and I'm just leaving for work. I wave goodbye to the kids, dump seven black bags outside ready for the bin men and begin the fifteen-minute walk to Clapham Junction.

Sue's hiding round the corner, peering over a bush and when the coast is clear she's tip-toeing like *Columbo* towards the house and having secret liaisons with assistant producers, designers and runners, all armed with tape measures and clipboards, deciding what theme they're going to go for in the living room and how they're going to transform the world's smallest bedroom into a space where three four-year-olds can exist without killing each other.

She had an extremely long to-do list, one item of which was knocking on all the neighbours' doors asking if they had any objections to the road being cordoned off, to cameras and catering trucks blocking up the driveways and to Peter Andre skipping about in a pair of dungarees. Luckily, they didn't. She also had to gauge if any of them would be willing to help out with the preparations. The two rooms that were going to be made over needed to be completely cleared before work could start. And then there might be bits of painting on the day that they could help with. She was met with a warm wave of positivity and a willingness to pitch in.

So the neighbours were in on it too. What sneaks!

Oh, and our choir mates. Little buggers! Sue obviously gave them very little choice. *This is what's happening. You're all on board. Spit spot – no time to waste!* Little did I know that emails were pinging back and forth, secret choir rehearsals were being planned and days off from work were being booked for the last Tuesday in April. I simply had no idea about any of it. Naive now, in retrospect. Of course something like this would involve a much wider group than the person lovely enough to fill in an online application form and press send.

Makeover Day itself came round with lightning speed and Mel whisked me away for twenty-four hours. I didn't make the connection initially. It certainly wasn't the first time in the last couple of years that she'd treated me to a night away or planned something lovely for us to to do but on this occasion the timing couldn't be ignored. Once the penny dropped it was a no-brainer that I needed to be safely out of the vicinity of home.

So, as the big day dawned, Mel and I woke up side by side in a hotel just outside of Watford. Her phone was buzzing and beeping from about 7 a.m. and I busied myself with my own mindless scrolling while she furiously texted and made whispered calls from the bathroom, emerging minutes later with her face flushed from the pressure of playing her part in making sure everything ran smoothly.

Another room, another elephant lumbering around. We kept catching eyes and either bursting into slightly hysterical laughter or saying in unison how sick we felt. We both made endless trips to the loo and neither or us had any kind of appetite at all, the delicious-looking hotel breakfast pushed to one side on our plates.

Back upstairs, tummies still empty, we flopped back on the bed for ten minutes before getting ready to check out.

There was a knock at the door and in the split second before it opened I couldn't resist.

'That's not Peter Andre, is it?'

Mel's face turned a deep shade of red, her shoulders dropped and her face crumbled. I wasn't quite sure whether she was going to laugh or cry.

'Oh babe,' she said, her bottom lip wobbling. 'It's been a fucking nightmare.'

It all poured out. The stress, tension and pressure. All stemming from a desire to do something amazing for me. Having to manage, from a distance, all the secrecy, fibs and organisational hurdles was enough to make anyone anxious.

Mel had been desperate to talk, to get it all off her chest. It was clear that there had been many points over the last few weeks where she'd wondered if she'd done the right thing. It felt good to reassure her that 100 per cent, without a shadow of doubt, she had. I was excited! I was grateful. I wasn't concerned about not liking what they might be doing to the house – how bad could it be?

It was one of the longest days of our lives. We just wandered around, killing time, waiting for the call to say that they were ready for us, that it was action stations.

As per instructions given to Mel from the producers, we met Miles in the pub two minutes from the house. Miles was there with a camcorder tucked out of sight under his arm. He'd been instructed to sit behind me in the car and film my reaction when we drove the short distance back to the house.

Miles got the final call to say they were ready for us. I felt sick. I think we all did. That's when the adrenaline really kicked in and it suddenly didn't matter one jot that I'd kind of known what was going on and that all day long we'd both been wondering if I was going to successfully fake a surprised reaction or whether my face would give the game away and ruin the whole thing.

All I can say is thank God I did know because I think if it had been a complete and utter surprise, well, I might honestly have fainted or vomited or just keeled over or something. It would simply have been too much for my brain and body to handle.

The close had been cordoned off. There were yellow bollards dotted around and a smattering of diehard Peter Andre fans stood huddled behind the red and white tape that ran along the side of the road. My heart was pounding and my mouth was dry.

As we slowly turned the corner the sight that greeted us was one I will never forget.

The first thing I saw was Rock Choir in full flow, belting out 'Mr Blue Sky', thigh-slapping actions and everything. There were cameras, lights and about a hundred neighbours and friends gathered round, cheering and clapping. Four or five big strapping handymen stood to the side as Mel stopped the car, I clambered out and Mr Andre himself appeared through the crowd.

He walked towards me smiling and pulled me in for a big hug. Everyone cheered, I was smiling so much my face ached.

There's a clip of my arrival on YouTube that makes me cringe, laugh and cry all at the same time. I climb out of the car and as I'm hugging Peter you can hear me say, 'I don't know what's going on, what's going on?!'

And of course I did know what was going on but I might as well not have because the shock and surprise felt so genuine, so unforced.

Peter took my hand and led me over to the house where Ella, Louis and Theo stood shyly with Mum and Lucia. Lucia had come to work with us when Connie had left two years earlier.

Lucia was yet another godsend, another angel. A very special young woman from Spain who showered the triplets with warmth and love and made my return to work at the agency possible. She stood there beaming, along with everyone else. Well, nearly everyone else. Where was Jake? I couldn't see him anywhere. Surely Jake was here?

Peter explained his absence. 'Jake felt a bit shy so he stayed with his grandad but don't worry, he's fine.'

Oh. My heart sank a bit. What a shame.

But there was Sue, beaming.

Sue! Suddenly it all made sense. Sue had gallantly stood in for Mel and been crowned most special friend for the day. I really did feel so loved in that moment. And so, so, so bloody lucky.

Filming is a slow old process as anyone who's ever been near a camera crew will tell you, so once my arrival had been captured we had quite a wait before we were allowed inside the house for the Big Reveal.

Peter was such a star, chatting to all the neighbourhood kids, taking selfies and signing autographs. He was just so bloody likeable, just as you would want him to be. Who you see on TV is who the real Peter is. Down to earth, genuine, likeable and just for the record he smelt bloody lovely too.

Moments before we were finally allowed to go inside, he pulled me to one side and whispered in my ear, 'Don't panic when you go in. I know you got a new sofa recently – well, it's safe; it's hiding in your neighbours' garage and you can put it back once we've gone.'

Oh. Okay. Phew. Thanks for the heads up, Pete. I had no idea what to expect. Would the walls be papered with tin foil? Would there be some kind of weird novelty theme going on reminiscent of the days of *Changing Rooms* and Laurence Llewellyn-Bowen? What if I hated it all and couldn't hide my horror? Oh sod it, it really didn't matter. The whole thing was just so flipping exciting.

Finally we got to go inside and it really was a wow moment. The living room had been completely transformed. The first things I spotted were two giant white fluffy lampshades hanging from the ceiling. They were definitely on the bonkers list, albeit fun and pretty inoffensive. There was new carpet on the floor; there was an orange feature wall with wooden crates as shelves which I absolutely loved; the legs of the wooden dining table had been painted and six brand-new white space-age-style chairs surrounded it. And my sofa had most definitely gone. In its place was an L-shaped sofa made out of wooden pallets.

Yes, you heard me correctly. Wooden pallets. It was certainly a look, that's for sure. They were padded and covered with about a million scatter cushions and actually, it was the kind of sofa that would have worked brilliantly in a conservatory or garden room but I could tell just by looking at it that it was not a squishy, sink-down-into-heaven sofa. Thank goodness Peter had given me the heads up because had he not, I might well have panicked.

The designer, Ben Hillman, was lovely and honestly, there were lots of aspects of the room that were gorgeous and very 'me'. The 'secret' pull-out drawers under the stairs made me squeal with delight – here was a place for all the plastic tat and broken toys at last! The room felt fresh and new and for the first time ever there was a place for everything. There were little thoughtful touches dotted throughout, including a blackboard up on the wall with wooden compartments for me to put pens and paper in. 'We know you love to write,' said Ben. My eyes filled up with tears. How amazing. On the blackboard was a scrawled message from Sue written in waterproof chalk that still remains to this day:

'This is all from people who love you xx'

I just about held it together.

And then it was time to take a look at the second room to have been transformed – the triplets' bedroom!

Ella, Louis and Theo could barely contain themselves as we followed Peter and Ben upstairs, accompanied by a lighting guy and cameraman. I was inwardly cringing at the thought of the terrible state their bedroom had been in when I'd last seen it the day before.

Broken blinds, cupboard doors hanging off, a bare lampshade and a jumble of dirty and clean clothes everywhere. To be completely honest, it was a bit of a disgrace. It was just so tiny for the three of them that I didn't know where to begin and it became easier to just shut the door and simply ignore the mess.

Peter slowly opened the door and the three of them ran in shrieking.

Wow.

Wow, wow, wow.

It was stunning with a touch of genius. Ben had taken inspiration for their bedroom from a retro sign that hung in our kitchen showing a Fab ice lolly. The walls were painted blue, pink and white and above each bed was a personalised wooden sign in the shape of a lolly stick. The three lightbulbs hanging from the ceiling had ice-cream cone shades and the rugs on the floor were made up of multi-coloured dots, to resemble the sprinkles on the top of the lolly. And just like downstairs in the living room, the new carpet, blinds and shelves made everything look so neat and clean.

Ella, Louis and Theo leapt from bed to bed whooping with delight. My heart was bursting. They deserved this, they really did.

Jake's absence was a real shame. I found out later that he'd been extremely distressed when he got back from school and saw the cameras, the crowds and strangers going in and out of the house with our furniture and belongings. After much cajoling from Sue, Miles and Grandad it was clear that he would be happier staying away, which of course was totally OK. I just felt awful later on when I heard how upset he'd been. He was in no way forgotten though. As we finished filming our reaction to the new bedroom there was one more surprise. Peter wheeled in a brand-new, bright red limited-edition bike, signed by Chris Hoy – a special gift for big brother Jake. It was all too much. What an amazing thing to have happened.

By the time all of the interior filming had been finished it was dark outside. Peter and the crew eventually left after a flurry of warm, effusive goodbyes and thank yous and the neighbours dispersed back indoors, all buzzing from what had been a truly special and completely unforgettable day on the close. Our wonderful close.

As beautiful as the two made-over rooms looked, the rest of the house was an absolute state. It looked like we'd just moved in, or were moving out – one of the two. The living room and triplets' bedroom had been completely stripped bare before the work started and every single thing had been stuffed into boxes and crates or left in teetering piles along the landing. I could barely get into my bedroom – there must have been twenty-five removal boxes in there. The adrenaline was slowly ebbing away and I suddenly felt completely exhausted and slightly panic-stricken. Thank God Mel was staying for the night and would be around to help for a few hours the following morning. We set to work, along with Miles, Sue and a couple of other friends, clearing, making space and creating some kind of order so that I could function until there was time to sort things out properly.

It was about half past ten when we finally got the kids to bed and took a seat around the refurbished dining table. The room looked stunning. Sue had ordered a Chinese takeaway and we opened some bubbly and raised a glass. There were more inadequate words of thanks from me before we devoured a feast of all our favourites: salt and chilli squid, prawn toast, noodles. We were ravenous, worn out, euphoric and all absolutely knackered.

My darling, soul sis Mel – what an incredible act of love from you to me. And Sue, wonderful Sue – who else could have made it happen like you? Look what you both did for me and the kids.

Thank you both. Thank you.

chapter twenty-nine
me and nicole

Blog Entry, September 2014, 'Where my Head's at…'

I'm torn. My three are hurtling towards the age of five with grubby knees from the school playground, a million priceless questions and spaghetti sauce down their jumpers. Jake has started secondary school and is on the brink of a whole new chapter. They are all still the centre of my universe and I theirs and for that I'm truly grateful but… there's a but and I'm trying to figure out what it is.

I'm mum, mummy and sometimes mumma and I love it. Occasionally Louis refers to me as 'stupid lady' but that's only when he's really cross.

They need me as much as ever and I most certainly need them. But something is missing. The balance has gone awry.

Is it wrong to admit that there's an increasingly large part of me that's fighting for some airtime? A part of me that wants to not just be mummy and remember what it's like to be Em?

As my trio are growing, I think I am too. Or changing or… something.

But how do I make room for something more? Is it wrong to even want something more? Shouldn't being 'mum' be enough?

The choir I sing in once a week is great for my spirits and a lovely break from the routine. The friends I adore keep me going and make sense of the world when all I see is chaos.

My health is good, I remain cancer-free and am no longer dealing with constant drama from a certain person. Life is good. I believe life can be great. I'm just a little restless, wondering what the final piece of the jigsaw might be.

I sometimes look at Ella, Louis and Theo and wonder how they got here. I mean, really… how is it that these three high-spirited imps have taken root so firmly in my heart but continue to challenge me like nothing else? What a different parenting experience to any that I've known so far with Jake. These three are wild and strong and noisy and yep, challenging. Really, really challenging.

Ours is not a calm and ordered home though I used to think I was calm and fairly ordered. Emotions are expressed at top volume, objects are thrown and tears are shed. Every single day.

I spend a lot of time thinking I'm getting it all so terribly wrong but then I look at them rolling around like lion cubs, falling off the sofa and into fits of giggles. I look at Ella reaching out to comfort Louis or Theo in a rare moment of softness. I look at Jake being the most incredible big brother and how much they all idolise him.

'I like you, Mummy,' says Theo at least once a day and I breathe a sigh of relief.

I like you too, Theo. I like all of you.

I guess we're doing OK…

And it's true. We really were doing okay – or at least I thought we were. We were getting there. Daily life was still full on, I was still juggling a million plates but it wasn't the same as before. There was a lightness now; I was starting to look ahead, look up, with just enough optimism to make a difference. I knew I was on the cusp of something more. I couldn't put my finger on what but I could feel it and I was excited.

Did you ever see that famous picture of Nicole Kidman? There's a grainy long-lensed paparazzi snap of her that went viral just after her divorce from Tom Cruise was finalised. Bare-faced, hair scraped back and eyes closed, fists clenched in what could only be described as a big, fat 'YES' moment. You could see it written all over her face. Relief. Freedom. Closure. If closure is ever really possible with the father of your children. But I recognised that feeling. As a result of court-enforced boundaries meaning that Marc and I would no longer be communicating, I felt as though the most enormous weight had been lifted. I felt safe, free and ready to fly.

So how do you approach dating when you've got four kids, wonky boobs, countless scars and more emotional baggage than you know what to do with?

It was extremely tempting not to approach it at all. To stay home, stay safe and wrapped up warm with no risk of rejection or scrutiny. The belief that no one would want to get involved with 'someone like me' was deeply entrenched. At what point when you're getting to know someone do you mention the cancer, four kids and crippling anxiety?

But after several excruciating attempts at creating some kind of online dating profile and the odd drunken night with Mel and Miles involving much hilarity while scrolling for possible suitors I finally bit the bullet. I paid a three-month subscription to eHarmony and dipped my toe into the world of online dating.

Not quite able to believe my courage, I sent a message to a guy called Peter. His profile picture had caught my eye immediately – the phrase 'silver fox' springing to mind as I zoomed in on his short grey hair and expensive-looking suit. After we'd exchanged half a dozen polite emails we arranged to meet for a coffee in Wimbledon on a Saturday afternoon. I had a choir workshop that morning and then I went for a quick bite to eat with the others before I left them to take the bus up the hill into the village.

I was incredibly nervous. Ridiculously so. I don't know what I was so afraid of but I was so far out of my comfort zone that I could barely breathe.

Finishing up my lime and soda at the pub, my lunch untouched, I burst into hot, angry tears. I felt furious! I didn't want to go on a stupid blind date; I just wanted to go home. It felt like a total waste of time and the only reason I didn't cancel was that at least once I'd done it no one could say I hadn't tried. I was sitting next to Linda – one of only a couple of friends who knew where I was headed – and she talked me round.

I'm sure you're not surprised to hear that the date was not remotely scary. That I was worrying about nothing. Peter was actually a really nice guy.

We chatted over coffee and, at Peter's suggestion, went for a drink at a pub overlooking the common. I had a coke – the early hour, an empty stomach and a wired brain would not have been a good drinking combination.

We chatted easily and honestly without getting too heavy, and after going through what I imagined to be the usual topics – work, kids, exes etc. – I took a deep breath and mentioned that I'd had breast cancer. I had nothing to lose, I wasn't sure if I'd ever see him again and it simply felt as though we were having a pleasant, polite chat. There was no need to be secretive about something that I'm normally happy to share with anyone.

He reacted in a measured, sympathetic way and I felt myself relax.

Woo-hoo! Here you are, Em. It's a Saturday afternoon and you're on a date. Get you! Who would have thought it, eh? You've had cancer, you've been on your own with four kids for four years but there is a life out there, a good life. Go get it, girl.

Or something a little less nauseating than that.

Imaginary voiceovers aside, I felt brilliant. Relieved. I'd survived a blind date. I'd been a grown up, an individual, a fully rounded person. Not incapable of relating to another man. Not damaged.

We met again a few days later. He suggested going for a drink and though I was unsure I said yes, having promised Linda I'd take her advice: 'If he asks and even if you're not sure, promise me you'll go on a second date. The second date is the one that will make it clear if there's anything between you.'

She was right. Over the course of the next few weeks, Peter wined and dined me and it was absolutely delightful, the best thing that could have happened.

Of course, me being me, I fell for him pretty quickly – ain't no such thing as casual in my world. He was easygoing, charming and had a definite twinkle in those steely blue eyes. He was successful, proactive and, having spent years with someone who'd never so much as booked a restaurant table in advance, it was a total joy to be taken to the theatre, to dinner on the Southbank, to be shown real interest, I guess. I lapped up the attention and all sorts of long-since dead and buried feelings flew to the surface. He didn't ever ask about the kids and I found myself not mentioning them much, which didn't feel entirely right, but hey, maybe that would come in time?

I could tell he was a ladies' man and I didn't think for one minute that he wasn't still online and clicking 'like' on the profiles of lots of other attractive thirty and forty-something women but I managed to compartmentalise my brain and just enjoy what we were sharing.

The last time I saw Peter was on a Tuesday morning back in Wimbledon.

I'd just had a routine, six-month check-up with Professor Powles. Not long to go before I'd be moving into the once-a-year category. I could not wait. One hospital check-up a year! Freedom from cancer was within my grasp; I could almost taste it, touch it and when it finally arrived I was sure as hell going to embrace it.

So nonchalant and relaxed was I about the appointment that I arranged for Peter to pick me up afterwards in the hospital car park on his bright red Vespa, the plan being that we would get a takeaway coffee and go for a walk on the common. Climbing on the back of his bike and feeling his hand on my calf as I wrapped my arms around his waist and our helmets lightly bumped was a moment. Were we about to take things to the next level? Maybe this day would be a turning point, maybe this guy with more freedom than he knew what to do with *could* take a chance on a bound and tethered woman like me?

We didn't get much walking done. We found a quiet, secluded spot and lay on the grass chatting. Chatting turned to kissing and kissing turned to other things. Not everything, but other things. I remember Peter lifting up my top and kissing my left breast. My soft, real breast. I remember not feeling embarrassed by the hardness of my reconstructed one. I remember feeling surprisingly confident as his fingers traced my faded, silvery mastectomy scars and his lips moved towards my fake nipple – the one that has no feeling.

I remember with total clarity, how pale and healthy my skin looked in the sunlight on that happy, sexy Tuesday morning.

The reason I remember it so clearly is that it was just a few short weeks later when the pale, milky skin of my left breast started to turn a bit pink.

And my one real nipple that Peter had also gently kissed on the grass on Wimbledon Common had changed, felt different, odd.

We were the most intimate we'd been so far and maybe that's why I felt a distinct shift as we stood up, brushed grass off each other's jumpers and slowly made our way back across the common. Maybe Peter had seen in my eyes that my feelings were growing. Maybe he didn't like my strange, wonky boobs. Maybe he had a date planned that night with a woman with no appendages. Maybe he just wasn't that into me.

Because by the time we'd walked back to the car park and I'd climbed on the back of his scooter it was clear that something had changed. A drawbridge had been pulled up and this man who'd put some colour in my cheeks and a sparkle in my eye had realised that he and I were not meant to be.

Sure enough, a few days later his *it's not you it's me* email came through and despite the brevity of our romance I still shed a tear or two.

We're at different stages... you've got small children... responsibilities.

He was right but I didn't want those to be the reasons.

Something buried so deep inside me had been woken up and I didn't want life to go back to how it was before.

Of course, I bounced back pretty quickly. On a level lurking just below the rejection, sadness and bruised ego was a feeling of trust in fate. Maybe it's an age thing. Maybe I have developed a little bit of wisdom over the years when it comes to affairs of the heart. If he didn't want to be with me then it must simply mean that we weren't meant to be and far better to find that out sooner rather than later.

Plenty more fish in the sea and all that malarkey. Well done, Em, at least you gave it a go!

The tears dried and very, very soon I had a spring in my step once more and a lightness of heart because I knew, I simply knew that someone amazing was coming my way.

Unfortunately, I didn't realise that amazing someone would have to share a space, share me, with something really rather grim.

chapter thirty

mirror, mirror on the wall... which is the pinkest boob of them all?

Blog Entry, November 2014, 'A Marvellous Mini Break...'

Don't you just love it when things come together? I've always found it very handy that my best friend lives up north. It means that every few months I simply have no choice but to gather together every scrap of available childcare and make a solo trip up to see her in Harrogate. It would be rude of me not to and I just know the kids wouldn't appreciate our endless chatting and wine slurping. Scrap that — the truth is I wouldn't appreciate them interrupting our endless chatting and wine slurping. Bad, bad mummy.

So, receiving an invitation to review Ox Pasture Hall Hotel just outside of sunny Scarborough was a no-brainer. Would I and a guest care to enjoy a complimentary overnight stay in one of their luxury suites with dinner and breakfast included... er, 'yes please thank you very much ever so kind of you don't mind if I do' was my cool, 'I'll just have to check my schedule' reply.

It took us about two hours to drive from Harrogate to Scarborough. With Mel at the wheel and me trying to ignore my pathetic passenger-induced queasiness, we arrived at our destination a little weary and definitely ready to relax.

We received the warmest of welcomes and were shown to our enormous suite — the honeymoon suite, in fact. There was more space than we knew what to do with, the rooms were tastefully designed and cosy with a huge bathroom that had the funkiest taps I've ever seen.

Tummies dictating the timetable as always, we wasted no time in heading to the lounge where a glorious pre-ordered afternoon tea awaited us. Glad that we'd purposefully missed lunch, we polished off freshly baked scones, sandwiches and cakes and took in our cosy surroundings while enjoying the heat from the wood-burning stove...

Another sign of things being on the up was being asked to write a guest review for a hotel in Scarborough. For a short while after the *Best* Bravest Women awards I had a weekly column in the magazine but still wasn't earning regular money from writing despite plugging away, blogging and being a columnist on a magazine for parents of multiples. I felt hugely motivated though, was using my time constructively at home and felt confident that paid commissions could soon be within my grasp.

Handily, Scarborough is up past Harrogate so I jumped at the offer, invited Mel as my plus-one and hit the road, leaving the kids some dry pasta and the contents of the freezer to nibble on for a couple of days. Ha ha.

Me and mirrors, just like me and phones, are not a great match. Not so much mirrors from the neck up: I enjoy the whole putting-on-make-up ritual in the morning and making myself look half human after a sleepless night is rather satisfying. No, it's mirrors and boob checking that has been another extremely dysfunctional relationship in my life in recent years.

I'm sure Mr Sharma didn't mean to cause such angst when he made a fairly throwaway remark once after a routine check-up way back during that first year of remission.

'Oh, if anything's wrong it'll show itself in your skin,' he said breezily as I put my bra and T-shirt back on while he scribbled notes in my records.

Er, thanks for that.

It was all I needed to hear. Those two words. Wrong and skin. That started right there the almost daily ritual of checking for something, anything that I decided might be construed as 'wrong'. God, no wonder I couldn't get my career off the ground

– the amount of time I spent looking for something frightening to latch onto and obsess about. There never was anything wrong, however hard I tried to find something. Until a few weeks before the Scarborough trip, that is.

The rash came on gradually. I don't know even know if 'rash' is the right word to describe the flushed, pale pink colour that seemed to be creeping around my lower left breast. Had it always been there? Maybe it had and I just hadn't noticed. That preposterous thought kept me going for a week or two. So fixated was I on the appearance of my breasts that I could have described their appearance while wearing a blindfold and with both hands tied behind my back. Or was it all the scarring from the attempt to make the left one the same size as the fake one that had taken its toll and was now causing a strange dusky hue? As wonderful a surgeon as Mr Sharma was, we hadn't had much luck in matching up the size of my boobs. Skinny and sick at the time of the mastectomy, he'd inserted an implant into my healthy breast to give it a little bit of, er, lift and to match it to my new fake breast. But then, rather annoyingly, I got less skinny and as my weight returned to normal my healthy boob got bigger and suddenly the imbalance was really noticeable. So more surgery followed; the implant was removed and he did his best to even things out a bit.

I didn't tell anyone about the rash at first. Kept busy, busy, busy. Four years clear, four years clear – tiptoeing into the fifth with delight and relief. So there simply had to be a non-cancerous reason for this subtle but unmissable change. There had to be. There absolutely bloody had to be.

I arrived for a night at Mel's house in Harrogate, the plan being that we would drive to Scarborough the next morning for our twenty-four-hour complimentary stay at the hotel. Mel, her husband Nick and their two girls had moved since my last visit and so this was my first stay in their new home. New house equalled new bathroom which meant new mirrors and a different light. It was an irresistible chance to check, check and check again.

'Just popping up to the loo,' I'd say every so often, interrupting our chat and probably leaving Mel wondering if I had developed some kind of incontinence issue.

I'd even flush the chain sometimes, just to make my far too frequent visits seems genuine. Up in the bathroom at the top of the house I'd lift my top and stare at my chest. I couldn't reconcile what I saw in the reflection with how I felt, which was fit, well, strong and, dare I say it, happy.

It didn't take long for me to tell Mel. I don't keep anything from her. Never have done.

'My left boob is looking a bit funny,' I said in the car the next morning as we set off to the hotel.

'Really, darling? What's wrong?'

'It's looking a bit red, has done for a couple of weeks. Don't know what it is. I'll show you when we get there.'

I think I sounded a bit nonchalant. Casual. Not too concerned. I was so desperate for it not to be anything serious that I just pushed it out of my mind, in between trips to the loo, that is.

The hotel stay was fun and we had a lovely time. Our bathroom was gorgeous which was handy considering how much time I spent in there, checking, looking, feeling and studying. I never did show Mel my red boob. We were too busy catching up, talking, laughing, planning.

I was happy. The kids were happy. I almost felt like life was on track. I almost felt like I'd made it.

chapter thirty-one
dave the who?

Our episode of *60 Minute Makeover* was aired on the last Tuesday afternoon of November – seven long months after the day itself. It was 2014 and just over a week before the triplets' fifth birthday.

I was beyond excited. The kids and I couldn't wait to see it and I'd planned the day carefully, inviting neighbours in for the live 2 p.m. post-*Loose Women* screening.

Sue arrived with bubbly and other lovely friends and neighbours brought home-made soup, fresh bread and cheeses. It was a mid-week, mid-afternoon daytime party! The kids were at school and very cross to be missing it but I'd promised them screening number two that evening with pizza and popcorn. Dad and Ro would also come by then to watch it – the second of many, many viewings that would take place that week.

I was nervous as well as excited. I had no idea, of course, how the show had been edited, how we would all come across and how our story would be told.

I needn't have worried. I was thrilled with the episode. It was beautiful. I didn't feel at all exposed or invaded, aside from one or two scenes of horror when Sue and Peter were rummaging through my overflowing cupboards or discussing the mortifying state of the triplets' bedroom.

There was even footage of me at singing at Abbey Road with the choir – filmed secretly without me having a clue! My life, our life had been captured beautifully: moving, tender moments blending perfectly with scenes of silliness amongst Peter and his team of handymen and women.

So, that was it then. Makeover done! It was all over. But there was no anti-climax. Instead I was left with a warm, soppy, rather gooey feeling inside. The world was a good, good place. People were good. There were happy stories to be told, happy stories with happy endings. I was proud of our story and proud of how it had been told. I just wished we could go back and do it all over again.

Ah well. Back to normal life. Our fifteen minutes of fame were over but it had been a whole lot of fun.

There were lots of messages going back and forth that day. I responded to a few tweets and 'liked' various comments on Peter Andre fan feeds and found myself following the *60 Minute Makeover* Twitter account. I was drawing the whole experience out for as long as I could.

So, that evening, when a direct message came through on Twitter I was happy to briefly 'chat' with a man who seemed to go by the name of Dave the Carpet.

Hi Emma, never got the chance to say hello on the day, loved doing your show – it was one of our favourites! Hope you're well. Take care, Dave x

Aww, how lovely. How nice to have one of the crew reaching out to say hi. I had no idea who this 'Dave the Carpet' geezer was but it was definitely sweet of him to get in touch.

His second message followed quickly on from my polite but brief reply to his first.

Hope you got rid of that awful sofa made out of pallets!

Two smiley face emojis followed.

I clicked on Dave's profile. Maybe I'd recognise him from the makeover day.

Bloody hell. It was him. It was him!

The hairs on my arms stood to attention. It was only bloody him!

I had spotted Dave on TV years before we met.

I don't remember what I was doing when I caught five minutes of an episode of *DIY SOS*. Maybe I was feeding one of the babies. Maybe Marc had just left after a row. Maybe a shelf had fallen down or another fuse had blown or maybe I was simply wondering if I'd always be alone.

It didn't feel like a life-changing moment at the time. I just glanced at the screen and there they were – the handymen. Half a dozen guys hard at it under the watchful eye of Nick Knowles. Putting up shelves, drilling holes in walls, all the while racing against the clock to get that episode's build completed in time. Black trousers, white T-shirts. Busy working. *Grafting.* For some reason my eyes fell on one of the men in the group. He had greying hair that had a slightly Paul Hollywood-esque look about it and bulging, tattooed biceps.

That's the kind of guy I need.

And not for his 'inked guns', strong jaw and extremely broad shoulders. I wasn't having my very own hideous Diet Coke Break moment. My loins weren't tingling with longing or desire. Desire? What's that? I was so switched off in that department that it would have taken a whole lot more than a split-second look at a middle-aged man laying carpet to get me going.

It was the idea of being with a man who did stuff. Who was capable. Who had a little bit of oomph and who might know what he was looking for in aisle ten at Homebase. And yes, yes, I'm well aware that we're living in an age in which I should be more than capable of doing my own DIY, but give me a break. Doing everything alone all the bloody time is exhausting. Emotionally, physically and mentally. It was the thought of having someone to lean on, just a little bit. Asking for help all the time and feeling so dependent was horrible and feeling so ill-equipped to cope with so many aspects of my life was really rather worrying.

Of course I didn't think any of these things in detail when I caught a glimpse of the guy who I would later know to be the handyman legend that is Dave the Carpet. It was just a very subtle, fleeting 'clocking' of a man hard at work.

He'd registered. Somewhere, in my subconscious, Dave the Carpet had made his mark.

chapter thirty-two
rudolph can take a running jump

Bloody Christmas Jumper Day. Wear a festive jumper to work and put a pound in the box for charity. All well and good but can't I just donate a fiver and give the novelty jumper side of things a miss? I've got to be careful with woolly jumpers. Broad shoulders and the aforementioned extremely asymmetrical boobs ain't a good combo. Oh, and I think I'm ever so slightly scarred from when I was a plump teenager up in Stornaway, along with my waif-like sister. Auntie Annie told me she had some jumpers she'd knitted going spare. Jumpers that were clearly created from a 1959 knitting pattern she'd found under the floorboards. She offered them to me because apparently she and I had the same kind of build. Fabulous.

Auntie Annie was delightful but not exactly what you'd call dainty. Not that I needed or wanted to be dainty. Just not such a big, strapping lass, which is exactly how I always felt up there next to my teeny tiny sis. I politely declined the jumpers and made myself feel better by eating as many Tunnock's teacakes as I could get my hands on.

So, the prospect of Christmas Jumper Day wasn't really floating my boat. But – reluctantly and also to avoid letting the side down at work – I gave myself a talking to, nipped down to Primark and purchased the last Yuletide sweater in the store.

Once at work the day started like any other – opening up reception, logging on, checking emails etc. I liked the slow start of a Friday. Agents and assistants would make their way into the office in a leisurely fashion at around 10am, coffees or ginger shots in hand, all happy to have made it to the end of the week.

The rash on my chest was still there and clearly getting worse by the day but I'd had blood tests and a chest x-ray the week before and the consultant dermatologist at Parkside had given me a course of antibiotics which surely would clear it up. I was due back at the hospital that evening for a follow-up. It would be all be fine. Everyone was telling me it would all be fine so that meant it would be, right?

Dave the Carpet and I were in full texting flow by now. We hadn't yet taken the enormous step of talking on the phone but the messaging was gathering real momentum with morning and night-time texts coming thick and fast. Our humour was clearly in sync and the light-hearted but decidedly flirty banter was increasing daily. Just like the rash on my chest.

Clients came in for meetings, all commenting on our silly jumpers, the postman arrived with several bags of mail and the accounts department deposited about a thousand remittances on our desk that needed stuffing into envelopes. The morning was ticking along and it was nearly time for lunch. Lurking under Rudolph's brown bobbly eyes the rash was bothering me but, as the uncrowned Queen of Living with Dark Thoughts, I was doing a reasonable job of keeping my mind on other things, like Dave and what snacks were on offer in the post room.

My colleague Terry was deep in conversation with a particularly chatty client but apart from that, reception was quiet. Unusually for me, I left my mobile phone on the desk when I popped up to go to the loo on the first floor. I came back down again a few minutes later. Terry and the client were still chatting. I had no idea as I was flushing the chain and washing my hands that my life was being casually turned upside down. Again.

(THIS is the reason I have issues with my phone. THIS is the reason I have some weird, fucked-up relationship with the object that should simply be a device to let loved ones know you're running late or a convenient way to book a table at your favourite restaurant. Phones should NOT be allowed to do this. They should not. I'm sure Steve Jobs and co's vision for the iPhone wasn't for it to be a bringer of doom. First I was tethered and tied to it with Marc and then with cancer, always waiting for bad news to come, to bring my world crashing down.)

Anyway. I sat back down, glanced at the screen and my stomach dropped.

Two words on my most hated list.

Missed call.

I hate missed calls.

Missed call and voicemail message.

I hate missed calls and voicemails. They make me shake.

The next words I saw made me dizzy.

Parkside Chemo Ward.

Parkside Chemo Ward?

I hadn't set foot in Parkside fucking Chemo Ward for three years. What the hell?

The room spun a little bit. Terry and the chatty client's voices faded away as my finger pressed play.

Hi Emma! It's Mel here from Parkside Chemo. Can you give me a call please? Thanks, Emma!

I actually thought I was going to be sick.

Why? Why did Mel from the chemotherapy ward need me to call?

Why?!

I didn't *want* to call her. I didn't want to press call on the stored number and hear a nurse pick up and distractedly mumble 'Parkside chemo' as she scrolled down her computer screen and wondered if she could last till lunch without dipping into the biscuit tin.

There's only one Mel I ever want to call and it definitely wasn't this one.

I had no choice though. Clearly. You can't ignore a call like that. You can't erase it, make it disappear. You're cornered, trapped. Christmas Jumper Day was over. An unflattering, shapeless jumper was no longer something to give any kind of energy to whatsoever.

I phoned the hospital. They needed me to go in and redo my bloods.

Why, Mel, why do you need me to come in and redo my bloods? You did them all last week, didn't you, Mel? The dermatologist requested a full blood count so they were done, weren't they, Mel? So I'd know, wouldn't I? I'd know if there was a problem that might be cancer?

'We just want to redo your tumour markers. I'm sure it's nothing to worry about. Can you pop in today? When can you get here? How soon can you get here?'

As soon as I can, Mel. I'll get to you as soon as I can.

I felt like my chest was going to explode as I walked upstairs to Thea's office and told her I had to leave work for the day. She said, 'Of course, go, don't worry, just go. It'll be nothing. It'll be fine. It's good that they're checking things out. You'll be absolutely fine, lovely. Let me know how you get on.'

I rang Dad as I left the building and asked him if he could pick me up at the station and drive me to the hospital. 'They need to see me as soon as possible, Dad. They need to redo my bloods. Something's wrong, I know it is.'

When I climbed into Dad's car he said all the right things, of course he did. He squeezed my hand again like he always does. We pulled in to the hospital car park and moments later, as I walked into the chemotherapy ward for the first time in years, I honestly think I could hear my heart breaking.

It was like I'd never been away. I could barely bring myself to look at anyone. I couldn't look at the familiar faces of the nurses who had once cared for me so beautifully. Ivan, Mary, Eileen, Mad Julie with the Novelty Socks — I didn't want to look at them because I didn't belong there on that Friday afternoon. I was supposed to be at work, answering the phone, greeting clients and franking the post and counting down the minutes until 'wine o clock' at 5 p.m. because that's the kind of brilliant company I worked for and because life was really, really starting to feel good. That's what I was supposed to be doing.

A nurse took my bloods and afterwards Hospital Mel (not *my* Mel) took me into a side room to look at the skin on my chest. The angry, red skin that was hot and itchy and swollen.

'Lymphoedema. I think it might be lymphoedema,' she said and the clouds briefly parted.

'Really?' I said as I slid off the couch and put my bra back on and pulled Rudolph over my head and then smoothed down my hair which Rudolph had made static as if I didn't have enough problems.

As I left the hospital I held onto lymphoedema as being the possible cause of whatever was wrong. I held onto the theory that a blockage of the lymph vessels causing an accumulation of fluid was what was making my skin red and tender and puffy. Lymphoedema was common after breast cancer, after surgery and lymph node removal. I'd always worried about having it but now I'd welcome it with open, swollen, arms if that's all it was.

Back at Dad's I walked straight upstairs to the spare room at the top of the house while Ro made tea and mother-henned me like no time had passed since the last time I'd needed clucking around.

I fell into a deep, deep sleep (mild narcolepsy kicking in as it often does when my stress levels soar) only to be woken shortly after by the phone ringing.

It was the hospital again. Fuck.

'Hi Emma, can you come in and see Prof this afternoon?'

It was Professor Powles's secretary, Hilary.

'Er... OK,' I replied, disorientated and instantly devastated that I'd been woken from the protective bliss of sleep and that this was my reality. 'What time should I come in?'

'As soon as you can would be good.'

I walked downstairs to the kitchen to where Dad and Ro were sitting looking sombre and talking, always talking. They looked up at me as I stood in the doorway, interrupting Dad's flow.

'Parkside called again. Professor Powles wants to see me as soon as possible. Can we go now? Please can we just go now?'

So we got back in the car and Ro came with us this time, letting me sit in the front passenger seat as she always does when there's a drama. I sat there like the Queen Mother with a rug over her knees and Ro told Dad to drive carefully and slowly and all I could feel was irritation and anger. Not at Ro and her kindness and softness but at my Queen Mother status. I didn't want to be driven like an ill person with an invisible tartan blanket over my lap. I didn't want to be on my way back to Parkside Hospital on Friday afternoon for an emergency appointment with my oncologist when I should be at work and not just on any Friday afternoon but Christmas Jumper Day Friday afternoon when I'm wearing a ridiculous jumper and a man called Dave the Carpet is messaging me and he's got no idea at all that any of this is going on and it all just feels so fucking unfair.

Back in the waiting room for the second time that day, Dave texted me.

How's work going? Are you going to send me a picture of yourself in your Christmas jumper then?

He signed off with three kisses and a cheeky emoji – the one with the tongue sticking out and one eye closed. You know the one.

I simply had no idea how to respond. All I could think about was how the events of this day meant that whatever might have been with Dave would be over before it had begun. And that made me so so sad because I was starting to feel little bubbles of excitement brewing. I was starting to feel happy that this man was sending me silly text messages and making me smile at random points throughout the day. He was starting to have an effect on me and I really, really liked it.

All I could think about was how if I lost Dave because of today, lost him before I met him because of the rash and the bloods and all of this... this... drama, then that really would be it for me on the love front. It really would be game over. Cancer's back so bye bye love. Who would step into that battlefield with me? Who would be mad enough to take on a love that was destined to be lost?

So I just made something up about it being a busy moment and that I'd send him a picture later. His thumbs up emoji response told me that he had no reason to think I was lying.

Prof called me in. I walked towards him, past the reception desk and he reached for my hand as he always did. His smiling face full of warmth and softness. It would be okay. Surely. Prof would tell me it was all okay, just like Dad. They were a similar age and Prof had become another incredible man in my life, another safe harbour. Another voice of comfort and reassurance. Until today.

Lying on the couch, naked from the waist up, like so many times before, he took one look at my chest and his face spoke volumes.

Such a wonderful man. How lucky I'd been to be under his care. How many times over the last four years had I sat in his office, my face white and pinched with fear. How many times had I lain on the couch while he expertly examined my breasts. How many times had he shooed me out with a peck on the cheek and a 'doesn't she look marvellous?' to Hilary or a 'isn't she doing well!' in a way that wasn't at all like Bruce Forsyth.

How many times has Professor Powles sent me on my way telling me to look both ways when I cross the road because he was more worried about me getting knocked down by the number 75 bus than dying from cancer.

But he didn't say that today. Unfortunately, not today.

Where are the Wombles when you need them? I could have really done with a hug from Uncle Bulgaria as we drove past Wimbledon Common on the way home. The common I used to love. The village, the open green space. Now, the village had lost its appeal and the common – the same common where in 1992 a young mother called Rachel Nickell was stabbed, sexually assaulted and murdered in front of her two-year-old son just looked sinister.

The news really wasn't great at all. My tumour markers had gone through the roof and, at closer inspection, the chest x-rays had revealed a shadow on my lung. I needed a biopsy, a CT scan and a PET scan as soon as possible.

The world had honestly never felt darker.

chapter thirty-three
alone but not

When I'm in a state about my health I find it hard to be around the children. My anxiety manifests itself in lots of different ways, none of which I'm very proud of. At worst, the fear makes me angry, incredibly irritable and horribly intolerant and at best it just makes me weep. Silent tears. Hardly the qualities that make for mother of the year.

Does avoiding my kids in the darkest of times make me a terrible mum? You'd think that I'd want to be around them even more. That I would want to sink to my knees, breathe in their smell and climb into bed with them all snuggled around me.

I can't handle it. I can't bear to look at their gorgeous, smiling faces. I can't bear Jake's ever-developing awareness which means that he inevitably picks up on something being wrong.

'Are you OK, Mum?' he asks when I have a look on my face that can only be described as stricken.

'Fine, darling. Fine,' I say, but I can barely muster up a smile. And so he skulks up to his room, closes the door and Ella, Louis and Theo start playing up because they can sense that I'm not present. But I'd rather that than see their joy because their joy makes it even harder for me to live inside my head with its constant thoughts of death and of leaving them.

So on the way back from the hospital, Ro rang Fiona to see if she was free to stay with the kids for the night so that I could hide away at Dad's.

Back up to the room at the top and back into bed. Was there anything else to do other than sleep? It was the twelfth of December. The triplets had just turned five. It was nearly Christmas. There were stocking fillers to buy, fairy lights to untangle and school plays to attend and I just wanted to scream and scream and cry and cry.

And there was Dave the Carpet too.

I needed to let him know how the day had unfolded. To explain why it had changed from being a day full of banter about stupid jumpers to short, uncharacteristically brief responses and then radio silence.

I didn't know how to word it. I didn't want to word it. It was almost as though by not telling him I could make it go away. His blissful ignorance somehow made a likely cancer recurrence less real. At about 7 p.m. he texted to let me know he was back from work. *How was the rest of your day? Didn't hear from you, was it busy? Hope you're OK x*

I took a deep breath, fingers shaking and tears streaming down my face.

My lovely Dave. Bad day here. Something has shown up in blood tests and I'm being sent for scans. I totally understand if you want us to stop talking. I feel such a connection with you but you don't need this and we haven't even met xx.

A few moments went by and then his response pinged through and it was completely in keeping with the man I felt like I was starting to know very well indeed.

Ems. I know this is a terrible day but we've connected for a reason. I'm going nowhere. I'm here for you. If you want me to be that is xx

And so we just kept messaging and evening turned to night and I pretended to Dad and Ro that I just wanted to be alone, that I was going to try and sleep. Ro stood at the bedroom door while Dad leant down and kissed the top of my head.

'That's good, my darling, you sleep and we'll see you in the morning. We'll sort all this out, OK? Sleep well, my angel girl.'

Dave held me tight that night, even though we were miles apart. He emotionally held me in a way I'd never experienced before and so when I finally drifted off to sleep in the early hours it was with a calmer mind than I thought possible.

chapter thirty-four
carrot cake and kisses

So is it too corny to say that I felt like I was driving towards my future on that cold, crisp sunny Saturday morning in December? The morning after the blackest of days.

Could that be true? It certainly felt like it. Driving towards a man I'd never met but who I'd briefly noticed on television years before. Who'd been in my house, laying new carpets, without my knowing. Who I'd been messaging back and forth for two and a half weeks and who already felt like the person I most wanted to talk to.

I'd barely slept. Dave and I finally stopped messaging in the early hours and started again at dawn.

Can I call you? I want to hear your voice.

And so finally we spoke and it was strange, funny, comforting and familiar.

'Can I see you today?' he asked. 'I know it's probably not possible but is there any chance that we could meet?'

And I simply knew I had to go. There was no time to waste. Whatever this was. Whatever was happening between us, I (we) needed to know so I (we) could face the next chapter.

I said yes knowing that I'd find a way of getting the kids taken care of. Surely someone would step in and let me go? Even if just for a few hours.

Dad and Ro crept in soon after. They peered round the door of the bedroom, clearly apprehensive about how they'd find me.

'How did you sleep, my darling?' asked Dad as he sat down on the edge of the bed and reached for my hand. His eyes were glistening as he sat there in his funny old towelling dressing gown with his hair sticking up at the back, exactly like mine does.

'Ro and I have been talking. Haven't we, Ro? And you're going to be fine. We'll get it sorted, my darling. We've been here before and we'll deal with it. You're strong – isn't she, Ro? Eh?'

It was those broad shoulders of mine, making me seem so much more resilient than I was, when in fact I don't think I'd ever felt so weak.

'We're confident, aren't we, Ro? Tell her, Ro – tell her how confident we are.'

I tried to absorb every word Dad said as I sipped the warm, sweet tea despite having learnt the hard way that there were some things even he couldn't put right.

And then, as his voice carried on, I stopped listening and began to feel like my head and heart were going to explode with the awful, awful timing of this fucking bollocks and suddenly, out of nowhere, I spluttered and crumbled and cried.

'I've met someone.'

'What? You're kidding! Have you?'

'I've met someone and he's lovely and we've been talking and I'm going to see him today.'

'Oh sweetheart,' said Ro. 'Who? Where? Who is he?'

Dad's voice quivered. 'Is he a good man? Is he kind?'

'He's from the makeover. He got in touch a couple of weeks ago and we've been chatting and he sounds so lovely and I've told him everything and –'

More tears came, of course they did. Jeez. Why can I never, ever do anything in a moderate fashion?

Five minutes after knocking on the front door of Dave's small but very cosy cottage in Surrey, I was standing in his kitchen shivering, coat still on, while he made tea. But not just any tea. He'd been out especially that morning to get Tea Pigs tea, the finest, most delicate little bags in the land.

You do drink tea, don't you? he'd texted a couple of hours earlier. I was briefly back at home at the time, doing my best to be in 'mum' mode while getting ready for something that felt a little bit like a date. But how could that be? A date?

And carrot cake? Do you like it?

My heart smiled at that last question. Not just because I love carrot cake more than most things but because it was a touching sign of his sweetness.

He'd bought 'special' tea bags and a carrot cake, just for my visit. Already, by far, the most romantic thing anyone had ever done for me. Ever.

We made small talk at the start, mostly about the only thing that linked us – *60 Minute Makeover*. Then midway through regaling me with stories of Peter Andre and the team, he stopped what he was doing and just looked at me. I smiled back and we both said nothing.

'Come here,' he finally said, putting down the milk jug and opening his arms. I stepped towards him and he held me close. And he felt so strong and I knew instinctively that I was safe and that, in that moment, I was exactly where I should be.

I didn't cry about cancer in front of him that day. I was surprisingly chipper, considering the dire straits I'd found myself in. We sat side by side on the sofa, TV on, drinking tea, eating cake. It got dark early and I made moves to leave. I wasn't really sure what I was doing. Should I stay, should I go? My kids were back at home; my family were holding the fort. I was sitting in a strange man's house. I was back in the horrendous limbo of knowing I was ill without being told outright and yet I also felt like I was on the world's strangest first date.

At about four o'clock Dave went to put a film on. It seemed like he wanted me to stay.

'Don't go yet,' he said. I was flagging, suddenly exhausted and confused. I wasn't sure what I was feeling but I knew I didn't want to go.

We sat back on the sofa and it felt right to lean into him, head on his chest. I could have slept like a baby and several times I felt myself nearly dropping off. Dave had chosen a comedy and kept laughing out loud, his big chest rising beneath me as I nestled in closer. I glanced up at him every so often, barely keeping up with the film, just taking comfort from the warmth, the candles and his arms around me.

And then, somehow, at some point, as Ben Stiller and Owen Wilson did what they do best and it really was time for me to go, we started kissing. Properly kissing. Passionately, frantically. It was absolutely amazing.

Wow. I had not expected that to happen. Clearly, neither had Dave.

'Je-sus Christ'! he kept saying every time we came up briefly for air before locking lips once again. 'Fuck-ing hell!'

'Stop swearing!' I said, even though I wasn't exactly giving Little Bo Peep a run for her money in the good behaviour stakes. I didn't recognise myself! 'Snogging' on a sofa with someone I'd only just met like a teenager and less than twenty-four hours after finding out I had cancer. Again.

I felt on fire. What was this? Who was this man?

After what seemed like hours but was probably only about forty-five minutes, we finally stopped and let me tell you it took a lot of self-control.

'I'll walk you back to your car,' he said as we stood in the middle of his living room, slightly awkward now that our bubble of intimacy had been broken. I glanced around the room one more time as Dave got his keys and jacket while his beloved ginger tabby Charlie weaved in and out of our legs. I felt at home here. The decor was familiar. Neutral colours, candles everywhere, an open fire – if I were sitting at home watching an episode of *Through the*

Keyhole I'd definitely be curious about who lived in a house like this. It was very 'me' and that felt good.

It was absolutely freezing outside and Dave gently put his arm around my shoulder as we walked slowly down the hill.

'Here I am,' I said, smiling shyly as we reached my car. The windows were already freezing up and Dave used the sleeve of his coat to wipe the front windscreen.

'Wow,' he said, peering through the glass towards the back seat. 'Three car seats!'

'Yeah,' I said, smiling. I was used to people's reactions to all the threes in my crazy world. Three babies, three toddlers, three seats in the buggy, three cots, three beds – once, twice, three times a baby.

I didn't know it at the time but that was a pivotal moment for Dave.

'I looked into your car,' he told me later, 'and saw three car seats in the back and it hit me, your situation, what I was potentially getting involved with.' But it didn't seem to put him off.

As first dates went – and I'd had tragically few – there was none of the usual *so, er... well, give me a call sometime, maybe we can go for a drink again.*

It was the strangest non-strange feeling I'd ever had. It all just felt so natural and I don't think there was ever a moment where either of us doubted we would see one another again.

'Give me a call later,' Dave said, kissing me softly one last time. 'And drive carefully, OK?'

As I drove off I could see him standing there, hand up in the air in a motionless wave, waiting until I was out of sight. He looked so strong, so stable, so rooted. What must he be thinking? Poor guy. His stress-free, simple life was about to get a whole lot more complicated.

chapter thirty-five
rock solid

Blog Entry, March 2015, 'Somewhere Between a Rock and a Better Place...'

And so I've hit the halfway mark. Four cycles of chemo down, four more to go. I'm sitting on the top of the mountain, catching my breath and hoping the descent will feel a whole lot easier than the climb. I'm doing well, according to my wonderful oncologist. The chemo is doing what it's supposed to do and I can see the visible proof. I'm saying 'thank you' quietly a thousand times a day.

Still got my hair. Yay. Well, most of it. This is a very nice, much appreciated bonus. It's shedding but slowly and I'm just hoping and praying that I don't wake one morning looking like Bill Bailey — shiny scalp and long straggly ends. Sorry, Bill — you wear it well but I just know I couldn't carry it off.

And yes, we've fallen fairly comfortably into our new routine. My amazing four seem to have adjusted to mummy's good and bad days without too much upset and the usual band of angels in my life are rallying around as I knew they would. I feel blessed. Knackered but blessed.

Something else is different too, this time round. Something completely unexpected but rather wonderful. There's a hand holding mine in the chemo ward. There's someone making me giggle uncontrollably as the hideous cold cap is being suctioned onto my head and I feel like I want to be sick, cry and scream all at once.

Chemotherapy and laughter were incompatible last time round. It was the loneliest feeling in the world. I've laughed more in the last three months than in the last decade. Who would have thought it? Definitely not me.

I've never had a rock before. Always cringed slightly at the word. Jealousy probably, or maybe more a feeling of not being able to relate at all to the idea of being able to lean into someone and exhale. I've had — I've got — other rocks, plenty of them. A super sister-shaped rock, a giant dad rock that's more like a boulder and more huge, shiny, rock-like friends than one woman deserves. But this particular type of rock is a first. And it's making everything better.

We don't talk much about cancer. He doesn't think of me as ill and therefore I don't think of me as ill. Best approach, don't you agree? Sitting in our corner of the chemo ward eating Maltesers and making plans is actually a pretty pleasant way to pass the time.

There's no doubt about it, cancer is rubbish but it could be worse, a whole lot worse and hey, spring is in the air. I plan to have a good spring. Let's all have a good spring. We deserve it, don't you think?

Dave and I were together from the start. Simple as that. From our first meeting at his house there seemed to be no going back, for either of us. For now anyway. He hadn't met the kids yet and, yikes, that would be the real test. Cancer? No problem. Three feral monkeys and an extremely attached eleven-year-old? We'd have to see. That was what was going on in my head anyway. Dave himself didn't seem worried. He seemed so robust about everything. So confident that we could rise to each and every challenge.

'We're going to look back on all of this one day,' he'd say as I sat, exhausted, in the chemo chair while he rubbed my feet.

'We've got so much to look forward to,' he'd continue as he talked about the places we would go and the things we would do when I was feeling stronger.

Looking back it's clear that I was in complete and utter shock.

'But I feel so well!' I kept wailing at the start. 'I don't understand how this has happened!' It got to the point where Hospital Mel actually shushed me as she walked past my chair and heard me babbling inappropriately to anyone who would listen.

I just didn't get it. I'd been exercising, juicing, running up the escalators on the way home from work. Running up the escalators at Waterloo station, for God's sake! If that isn't a sign of being in tip-top physical shape then I don't know what is.

I'd been feeling invincible and strong, emotionally and physically. And then chemo started and I felt like I was dying.

The cancer turned out to be a localised recurrence but I didn't find that out until much later because I was too scared to ask any questions. I also never really got to the bottom of the mysterious shadow on my lung – again because I was too scared to ask questions. For a good six months after re-diagnosis I was convinced that my medical team were keeping the really bad news from me. That they weren't telling me I had a secondary tumour in my lung. That's how my brain worked. How my brain still works. I used to sit in my chemo chair and watch the nurses talking at their station. Sometimes it seemed like they were whispering. I decided that they were whispering about me. It's a very, very exhausting way to live.

One thing I did know from the start of this new diagnosis was that my treatment would be long term. When the chemotherapy was over, and if I was lucky enough for it to have worked, I would then simply segue onto what oncologists call 'maintenance treatment'. Alongside the chemo I was being given two incredible drugs – Herceptin and Pertuzumab – and these are what I would continue to have, every three weeks, indefinitely. The aim was that the combination of these 'wonder drugs' would keep me in remission or at least showing no evidence of disease, which is how they tend to put it these days. Early on I did pluck up the courage to ask Mad Julie with the Novelty Socks how long I might remain on the treatment. Her answer was sobering. 'Well, normally, you'd stay on it for as long as it works.'

Oh. Right.

So that implies that it will stop working at some point then.

Some of those closest to me struggled with how adamant I was that I didn't want to know too much but this was and has always been my way of coping. I've said it before and I'll say it again – if there comes a point where I need to know certain things then I've no doubt that I'll be told. Until then, this is how I cope.

I'm not quite sure my relationship with Dave would have made it off the starting block if I hadn't been in the middle of cancer treatment and, as a result, had my incredible army of angels around me once more. You'd think that falling in love and then quickly embarking on an intimate and extremely passionate relationship with someone would be dramatically hindered by the misery of chemotherapy and potential hair loss, fear of death, etc. etc.

Not for us. Because I was ill my nights spent at Dave's house were considered to be (by those who rallied around so wonderfully) respite care. My small but incredible 'sleepover' team made it possible for me to stay over at Dave's house for a night or two, every couple of weeks.

Had I not been ill, how would I have justified this regular time away from the kids? How would our relationship have survived those delicate early days when time alone is essential?

Hotel Belmonte. That's what Dave and I called his house, naming it after Belmont, the village he lived in. I'd arrive on a Friday evening, weekend bag packed, and he would take my coat, lead me to the sofa, put a glass of wine in my hand, and kiss me on the lips before heading back into the kitchen to carrying on preparing dinner.

I didn't lift a finger. He cooked, washed up, ran me candlelit bubble baths and made it so perfect that, as much as I missed the kids, leaving was agony. In an ideal and sane world, Jake, Ella, Louis and Theo would have been with Marc every other weekend. I could have waved them off after school on a Friday or first thing Saturday morning, safe in the knowledge that they were with their other parent having a happy, safe, harmonious time. I could have legitimately switched off with no need for more guilt or feeling indebted to dear friends and family. If only that part of my life could be simple.

I would sit staring blankly at the TV or listening to the music belting from his state-of-the-art, dogs'-bollocks speakers and wonder how I'd got there. I'd lie in bed in the morning having had the priceless luxury of being allowed to wake up naturally and despite the strands of hair on the pillow or the ulcers on my tongue I would feel happy. Really, really happy.

How had this happened? Who was this incredible man who had turned my whole world upside down in the most wonderful, healthy way? Who had, in the shortest time, become my lover, my best friend, my confidante, my rock and, ultimately, my seahorse?

'We're seahorses,' Dave said one night as we cuddled in bed, arms, legs, feet wrapped round each other. Lionel Richie was playing on the radio, singing words of love that felt like they'd been written for us.

'Eh?' I said, looking puzzled. 'Don't you mean soul mates?'

'Nope. We're definitely seahorses. They mate for life. This is it for us. Well, it is for me.'

It certainly felt like our seahorse tails had entwined and that it was us against, if not the world, then cancer. I was the most joyful I'd ever felt but also the most scared. Life was dark and light. Two extremes. The most wonderful of times and the hardest. So maybe that's why I was so determined to enjoy my time with him, our times together at Hotel Belmonte, and to leave cancer in the pub car park at the bottom of the road, with the car.

Lust, sex, tenderness, laughter and a deep, deep connection – there was such an abundance of those ingredients in those early months with Dave that I'm not surprised I responded so well to the chemo. I was like a teenager. Except not Emma the teenager. Someone else entirely. Not the virgin in the corner who was simply incapable of communicating with, let alone getting naked with, boys.

What a wonderful, delicious, delightful distraction Dave was.

chapter thirty-six
my angels were back

Blog Entry, January 2015, 'An Unexpected Blip...'

Ella, Louis and Theo are thriving. Just turned five and quite possibly at the pinnacle of cuteness. They run into school each day smiling and happy and emerge a few hours later smiling and happy. They get home and they scream, they shout and it's still utter mayhem but it's our life and it's all been OK; we've managed to stay on track in recent months without too much casting a shadow. In fact we've had the sunniest of spells in years.

So, about now, I should be high-fiving myself for making it through. About now, I should be quietly celebrating my fifth of year of being cancer-free.

Turns out that I wasn't quite as free as I thought. And so, for the second time in my babies' little lives I'm embarking on the joyous journey that is chemotherapy. I'm bracing myself for three little horrified faces when they see me without hair for the first time. I'm preparing myself for six months of stepping back into the very much unwanted identity of an ill person, for a freezer full of lasagnes and kind gestures and, heartbreakingly, for my children to inevitably look at me in a different way.

Jake, my big handsome boy, is quietly shattered and struggling with the memories of last time, knowing what lies ahead. The little ones will simply be cross that very soon I won't look like mummy. I know this because of their reaction to the odd photo they've seen of that challenging time. The bald me of four and a half years ago – clutching my beautiful babies and smiling at the camera, attempting to appear like everything was tickety boo when really it was just rubbish. Really rubbish.

'I don't want that mummy,' said Ella a while ago as she studied the one picture of that time I have displayed at home.

I don't want to be that mummy either, darling. I'm so sorry, my angel. Do you know how much I love you?

Deep breath then and off we go. Another chapter for me and my four. As usual, they'll probably show me the way. They'll teach me how to 'be' – how to handle this latest setback. This was not part of the plan but I know there'll be some magic in it. There already has been. I know that we'll emerge from this even stronger and more resilient, even more full of love and appreciation for what we have as a family. I'll eventually accept that actually I look pretty damn good with a pixie cut and that when it comes down to it, nothing really matters other than the five of us being together with me being 'mum'.

The thing I moan about, the thing I struggle with, the thing that has felt so draining at times is now the very thing that will get me through, again. Being mum. The biggest motivator of all.

So come on then, cancer. I'm really trying not to take this personally. Let's make this latest visit of yours a quick one, OK? If that's all right with you? You can come in but please don't make yourself at home. There are five of us here with big, crazy plans and you're kind of getting in the way.

Sue stood up during a break at choir and addressed everyone in no uncertain terms.

'You've probably heard about our Emma. She's not well again and she needs our help. I've been to see her: the chemo is brutal, she's trying to look after the kids on her own and she's completely exhausted. To put it bluntly – and she'd be extremely cross if she knew I was saying this – she needs cash.'

It's true, I would have been mortified if I'd known Sue was going to make a such a bold request. But I'd be lying if I said I was in a position to turn it down.

There was a whip round and £500 was raised. Sue handed me a brown envelope. 'There you go,' she said briskly in her usual, no-nonsense fashion. 'Use it wisely.'

All I wanted to do was sleep. To be left alone to sleep. If money could buy that luxury then it was definitely a good use of my choir friends' generosity.

Katy gathered the troops once more and, just like before, they showed up, ready for action.

'We can make sure you have a cooked meal every night, would that help?'

I was tired, so tired I could barely answer the question. So much more tired than I could remember ever feeling before.

Lovely Tony from the choir's bass section bought me a chest freezer that we managed to find space for in the kitchen.

Kerry dropped frozen meals round.

Celia, Katherine, Dawn and her delicious chicken pie. Jo and her *I'm in Asda if you need anything* texts.

Sophie would turn up on a Saturday afternoon and load the dishwasher and cook the kids' tea and tidy up before she went. 'Sit down, Em. Just go and sit down.'

Wow. We really are back here then. Back in this needy, useless, dark, dark place. The only light seeping in through the cracks was from the hearts of those who surrounded me.

A microwave. I didn't like the things but when a lady I'd never met sent me one, having heard that I was struggling to cook properly for the kids, I wept with gratitude.

I was part of an online group of 'multiple mums'. We all had twins or triplets and all had a similar outlook on life – full to the brim with positive quotes and trying to live our best lives despite differing circumstances.

They wanted to help.

Can we set up a Just Giving account for you? Would you let us?

Oh God.

I deliberated and cringed and felt embarrassed and ashamed and didn't want to tell anyone about it. But it was either that or continue to drain Dad dry. At the start I'd hoped I might be well enough to do the odd day or two at work but it quickly became clear that the effects of chemo would scupper those plans. I got as much support as ever from work: the door was always open and they did all they could to make things easier, but it was the extra-curricular childcare that drained the pot dry. The times three-ness of everything. Three for the price of one, or even two, it certainly wasn't.

Last time round two very special old friends, Maria and Karen, got together and raised some childcare funds. They asked my permission before they emailed a long list of friends who they thought would want to help. I agreed, of course I did, but I found the whole thing torturous – I was terrified of being judged, my own voice of judgement roaring loudly in my head.

Shame is a horrible emotion but it's one I've battled with a lot. I felt deep shame that I was in this mess. That I didn't have a few thousand pounds in the bank to draw on until I was (hopefully) back on my feet again. All the giving, all the wonderful, kind, unconditional generosity was so incredible and so welcome but the cold, hard cash side of things was a tough one to get my head around.

My vaguely spiritual side believed that it was OK to accept, be open to what was coming my way, that the universe is fundamentally abundant and by accepting people's money I wasn't depriving anyone else of theirs.

They were my beliefs but the critical voice spoke louder most of the time. All that 'old' stuff from first time round came roaring up to the surface.

Look at the mess you've made of everything.

Look at what you've done. Take responsibility for your choices and actions.

Expecting everyone else to pick up the pieces again, are you? What a bitch. What a selfish bitch.

I said yes to the offer of a Just Giving account but it twisted my insides, made my cheeks flush and my toes curl.

'Accept, accept, accept,' said the lovely ladies so insistent on helping. 'Stop resisting and just let it in. You would do the same for us. We know you would.'

And of course I would and I knew they were right and I know I would have said exactly the same to anyone in a similar situation to me. Why do we find it so hard to accept help and still feel worthy and good about ourselves? It's cruel, really. If anyone spoke to Ella the way I've spoken to myself at times I'd take them down.

I'm stronger now. My self-worth and self-esteem has moved up the scale. But back then I was knocked out.

chapter thirty-seven
one last picture

Let me introduce you to Dave.

Dave is fifty years old and lives in Surrey. He runs his own carpet company and also appears regularly as a handyman on TV's 60 Minute Makeover. He has one grown-up son, George – a lovely, decent guy, just like his dad.

Dave has come through his own rocky times. He's survived a painful divorce and now lives happily alone with his beloved cat, Charlie. Dave has mellowed as the years have passed. He loves his work, keeps his house neat and tidy, is passionate about music (eighties soul) and one of his favourite things in the world is sitting in his pants with a nice cold beer and watching the footie on his huge, state-of-the-art TV.

Oh dear.

Oh dear, oh dear, oh dear. Dave, Dave, Dave. What have you done?

I was really worried about Dave meeting the kids en masse, for fairly obvious reasons. Not because they aren't great kids, not because they are essentially unloveable or, God forbid, unlikeable. But simply because there are so many of them. It was an enormous step in our relationship and we both knew how important it was to get it right, for everyone's sake.

We started the whole process gently by adopting a one-step, one-child-at-a-time approach. A gradual easing in for Dave and hopefully a fun introduction for the kids.

We picked a low-key, family-run Italian restaurant in yep, you've guessed it, Wimbledon. And once a week, for a month, I took one child to meet Dave for an early evening meal of pizza, ice cream and whatever the hell they fancied.

It was Jake's turn first. He was eleven and very aware that Mummy had met someone – mainly, I suspect, because of the time I spent glued to my phone. Some days he seemed okay with it and some days definitely not, which was totally understandable. It was a lot for him to take in. Again. Just like the first time when almost overnight he'd gone from being an only child with two together parents to the older brother of three squawking babies with a sick mummy and a very upset and angry papa, not to mention having to deal with a house move too. This time round, older and much more aware of what it meant to have cancer, and having just settled into secondary school, it was another miserable blow for my beautiful boy.

He had every right to be unsettled and anxious. To be clingy and demanding.

Why do you have to go out, Mum?

Where are you going?

What time will you be back?

Why is Nana sleeping over again?

I hate you, Mum. You're mean.

I love you, Mum. I miss you.

Was I wrong to take up Mum's incredibly welcome offer of sleeping over at the house so that I could go and stay at Dave's? Even if I was, I'm not sure that would have stopped me. Falling in love, as well as making me happier than I thought possible (cancer aside), also made me selfish. Surely I deserved this joy? Surely it was OK to say yes to the universe again and go with the magic that had come my way? Did it make me a terrible mum? Did it? The guilt, always so much guilt. My tumour of guilt that does not, will not, respond to treatment.

So of course I took up Mum's offer to sleep over and Miles's offer to have the kids at his place for the night. I just said yes, yes and yes again. The good news was that I needed less practical help this time round; with the kids at school I could rest in the day, something so desperately lacking first time round. There were many, many days when I would curl up on the sofa at 8.45 a.m. and not move until 3 p.m. I felt absolutely obliterated by the chemotherapy this time round.

Or maybe I was so exhausted because on the weekends that I saw Dave we spent pretty much the entire time in bed, doing anything and everything other than sleep. Somehow, don't ask me how, I always managed to summon up the energy to go to his house, looking reasonably OK, and to put my illness somewhere. Just for twelve or twenty-four hours. I was determined. Cancer was not going to stop me enjoying every single second of falling head over heels in love. Cancer was not going to stop me having the best sex of my life and cancer was certainly not going to get in the way of me feeling like my whole world had just opened up.

Falling in love and cancer. Talk about contrast. Chemotherapy and the Kama Sutra? Not a match you'd imagine.

So one child, one pizza and unlimited ice cream, once a week for four weeks. Simple. It went pretty well. I could see the relief flood across Jake's face within seconds of meeting Dave.

'Hello mate, how are you?' said Dave, extending a hand out to my biggest, but still so tiny, boy.

'Fine, thanks,' Jake beamed back, looking more like Harry Potter than Daniel bloody Radcliffe. Dave walked ahead of us into the restaurant.

'I like him, Mum! He's really nice!'

Oh thank God, Jake. Because I like him too. I really, really like him.

The week after it was Louis and it went as smoothly as clockwork. Then Theo, yep, no problems. And finally, my tricky little missy – Ella.

It took a while with Ella. She's no pushover, for which I am truly grateful and incredibly proud, even though as she fidgeted on her seat and didn't like her pizza and screeched for more apple juice I kind of wanted to strangle her.

First tentative meeting with each child done. Phew.

The next step? Dave being in the same room as all of us. All of them. At the same time.

I clearly wasn't of sound mind when I suggested he come over one Sunday towards the end of February. We'd been skirting around the subject for a while and I was letting Dave lead the way, allowing him to give me the nod when he felt that he was ready to take that next gigantic step.

'I think it might be time,' he said one night during our regular bedtime phone call.

'I've got a good idea!' I piped up excitedly. 'Why don't you come over on Sunday and spend the day with us? We'll just have a cosy day, we can snuggle up, watch a film. I'll make a nice lunch. It'll be fun!'

THERE SHOULD HAVE BEEN AN INTERVENTION.

Someone should have stopped me.

What the hell was I thinking? A cosy, snuggly Sunday with three restless, hyperactive and utterly defiant five-year-olds?

I nearly lost him. I nearly bloody lost the most amazing man I'd ever met.

Dave was confident in the days leading up to Sunday. He was unbroken, strong, untarnished by the triplets' reign of terror.

How hard could it be? he thought.

'Kids love me!' he said.

'Mum always said I should have been a children's entertainer,' he boasted confidently.

Well, I'm sorry, my darling, but even Mr Tumble might have struggled on the day that came to be known as yep, you've guessed it, Black Sunday.

It was raining, pissing it down, which meant the day was pretty much a write-off for me from the very start. The kids had woken up before 6 a.m. and by half nine I was already completely shattered.

Louis was in super anxious mode, Theo was being thug of the week, Ella was screeching and squawking like a mini Margaret Thatcher and Jake was winding them up into a frenzy. I desperately wanted it to be a perfect day. I wanted him to fall in love with them and them with him — just like I had. I wanted us to show him that we were the perfect family, even though we weren't. Had I learnt nothing in my eleven years of being a parent?

I'd had chemo that week so wasn't feeling my best but had washed my thinning hair and put on what I hoped were some casual and cosy clothes which would show me to be the perfect blend of cool mum and sexy girlfriend. Yeah, right.

Dave arrived at about half ten. The kids were slumped in front of the telly, slack-jawed and uninterested. The biscuit tin had been emptied, the cushions were strewn all over the floor and the washing machine was doing its about-to-take-off super spin thing which meant that the paper-thin walls in our paper-thin house were shaking and the windows rattling.

'Guys!' I said with a manic cheeriness reminiscent of Floella Benjamin at her perky *Play School* best. 'Dave's here! Remember Dave? Mummy's friend? He's come to spend the day with us and we're all going to have a lovely time!'

They didn't look up. Ella was sucking on her stinky rag, Theo had his finger halfway up his left nostril and Louis's right hand had found a warm and snuggly place down the front of his trousers. Jake was upstairs but that was OK, he'd come down in his own time.

'Tea! Let's have tea! I'll put the kettle on!'

Dave took his coat off and got stuck right in. I had to hand it to him: he gave it his all, without being creepy and weird of course. Short of juggling hoops and producing a live white rabbit out of a hat I'm not sure what else he could have done to make a positive impression.

Ella was incredibly wary and wouldn't go anywhere near him, carrying on with the ice queen vibe she gave off at the restaurant. Theo was mildly amused at his jokes and silly faces but more interested in watching back-to-back episodes of *Horrid Henry* and Louis was just being Louis. My little ball of stress.

OK, well, it wasn't a spectacular start but at least it was calm. So far so good. Ish.

And then Dave offered to help put together two Ikea bathroom drawer/storage-type things for me – they'd been lying in a corner of the living room for weeks, obviously unopened. My heart expanded even more. He got his toolbox out of the van and I made a space in the middle of the living room. The TV was still on in the background and the kids seemed pretty content.

Until he set to work.

'What you doing?' asked Theo suspiciously, sliding off the sofa, at which point Ella and Louis looked up and followed suit.

'Putting this together for Mummy,' he replied as the three of them gathered round, staring at him. 'Would you like to help me?'

Such an innocent suggestion. Such a potentially lovely activity for everyone to get involved in on a cosy, family Sunday.

Who would have thought that Ella being allowed to turn an allen key two times more than Theo would cause the whole house of cards to come falling down? Who would have imagined that three floppy-haired terrors all vying, jostling for prime position next to Mummy's friend Dave and his Black and Decker drill could cause such carnage?

'My turn, MY TURN!' screamed Theo, shoving Ella so hard that she flew backwards and hit her head on the coffee table. Cue glass-shattering screams.

'Theo, stop it! That was naughty!' I shouted, my face twisting into its default angry, furrowed expression as I pulled Ella up off the floor and gave her a token cuddle while trying to intercept where the next blow might be coming from.

'My go now! *It's myyyyy tuuuuurrrrnnn!*' screamed Louis, punching Theo on the back and then throwing a toy train at his head.

Dave was phenomenal. He kept calm and in control. Within five minutes he was crawling around the living room on his hands and knees being a monster and the kids were in hysterics. The boys were, at least. Ella was having none of it.

'Get away from me!' she screamed every time he came within ten steps of her.

'Nicely, Ella!' I'd say through gritted teeth and with a clenched jaw while she gave him her most ferocious stare and I gave her mine.

Lunchtime was hell. Picky bits! I'm famous for them. If in doubt, out comes the hummus, pitta bread, maybe a bowl of crisps or two. Carnivore Dave politely nibbled on an uninspiring salad and dipped a carrot baton into a tub of taramasalata. The kids were a flipping nightmare.

Breadsticks went flying across the room, plastic beakers of apple juice cascaded onto the floor and Louis had the mother of all meltdowns because Ella had the audacity to take the last Hula Hoop. It was clear Dave didn't know what had hit him.

Clearing up the debris after lunch, we found ourselves briefly in the kitchen on our own. We had a hug.

'Are you OK?' I asked tentatively, bracing myself for the worst. He looked ashen.

'It's full on, isn't it?' he said as tactfully as he could. 'How do you do it? I've only been here a couple of hours and I'm shattered!'

My heart sank. I could read between the lines. This was an absolute disaster. What was I thinking? Whatever had possessed me to make the poor man suffer an all-day-long visit to his cancer-stricken new girlfriend's house to meet her children properly, in their own environment – an environment utterly devoid of consequences, structure and discipline?

The saving grace was that Fiona and Mum were coming round later for dinner, along with Jasmine and Joe, my niece and nephew. By the time they turned up at the end of the afternoon I was struggling to hold it together, convinced that Dave would be running for the hills before pudding was served.

Fiona couldn't wait to meet Dave. Mum was understandably wary at first but once Dave gave her one of his epic hello hugs and she found out that they shared a love of shopping in Lidl, that was it – it was love at first squeeze.

We finally got Ella, Louis and Theo to bed about 8 p.m. Mum had made an early exit as her Sunday evening TV viewing was all meticulously planned out at home and Jake and Joe were upstairs doing whatever boys of a certain age do.

Dave and I sat side by side, opposite Fiona and Jasmine. The living room was restored to order, my trusty candles were flickering on every available surface and soft music was playing in the background. This was more like it. This was lovely! Fiona and Dave had hit it off instantly, Jas was bonding with him over a deep love and encyclopaedic knowledge of music and I kept looking at him thinking how right it felt that he was there, by my side. We were back to being us. Loved-up Dave and Ems. We both nervously giggled as we talked about the madness of the day and I had to stop myself from leaning over and kissing Fiona as she did such a fantastic job of trying to paint a more balanced picture of my life with the kids.

'They're not always so badly behaved,' she said, attempting to reassure Dave. 'They're great kids. And they're only five, it's going to get easier.'

'You two look so cute together,' said Jasmine as she picked up her phone to take a photo. Dave put his arm around me and I nestled in. I felt a lump rise in my throat. I felt sick. My bottom lip wobbled.

Hold it together, Em. Hold it together.

'Go on then,' I said. 'Take one last picture of us together.'

The three of them looked at me.

'Em!' said Fiona.

'What are you talking about?' said Dave.

'Well obviously, after today, that'll be it. We won't see you for dust.'

Dave looked at me and shook his head. He squeezed my hand and smiled.

'Don't be silly,' he said softly.

But I wasn't convinced. Ours was a madhouse and today he'd seen us at our worst.

I climbed into bed that night feeling drained and very, very flat. Dave called to let me know he was home safely and to say goodnight. Our conversation inevitably turned to the events of earlier.

'I'm not going anywhere,' he said. 'But if we're going to make this work then you and I need to be a team. The kids are great but they're running rings around you and it's hard to watch. I've actually never witnessed anything like it and I work in people's houses every day. I can help, if you want me to.'

He was so right. They did run rings around me. Somewhere along the way I'd got stuck. Stuck in survival mode, always looking for the easiest way to get through the next ten minutes, the next hour, the half-term holidays with no back-up, trying to deal with the off-the-scale tantrums, the unrelenting exhaustion. My parenting mantra was simple but way off track: *just do whatever the hell it takes to get through.* Give in; give them what they want; say yes, yes, yes when you should be saying no, no, no. Yes to another biscuit and oh all right then to no more carrots. I was scared of saying no. Scared of being consistent, getting tough with four kids who clearly needed boundaries. Scared of the repercussions. Scared of them.

It was time for me to take control of things at home. For the kids' sake, for my sake, for my fragile new relationship's sake. I couldn't risk losing him. Being alone again, being without Dave was something I couldn't bear to think about.

chapter thirty-eight
a fumbling fairy tale

By the end of 2015 and within a year of us getting together, Dave had sold his house and moved in to mine and together we had an ambitious and exciting plan to extend it and make it 'ours'.

There were always going to be concerns from those on the outside looking in.

Are you sure, mate? asked his friends. *I know you love her and everything but bloody hell, four kids? Cancer? What are you going to do if it doesn't work out?*

Do you really want to take someone on with so much baggage? Do you really want to start all over again?

What if the cancer comes back again? Then what? Think about it, Dave.

I'm pretty sure he did think about it. Endlessly. There must have been many a night when Dave lay awake wondering what the hell had happened to his sane and steady life. Maybe it was the circumstances of our meeting that set the fast and furious pace of our relationship.

Maybe, if cancer hadn't been part of the picture, we would have dated for a while and then drifted apart as the demands of our very different lives took their toll. Maybe we would have fallen just as deeply in love but struggled to make it work because I wasn't free like he was.

Cancer brings everything into focus. Maybe cancer's gift to Dave and me was clarity.

A couple of months before he moved in, Dave arranged for us to have a night away at a beautiful hotel near Egham in Surrey. It wasn't a birthday or special occasion and as I packed my overnight bag and made sure everything was in order at home I thought about how much I loved that side of him. He thought nothing of planning random surprises, booking theatre or concert tickets just so that we always had something lovely to look forward to.

'We deserve it,' he'd say and slowly I was starting to believe him. I began to give less airtime to the negative chatter that told me I was a bad mum for taking time out. That having fun and good times away from Jake, Ella, Louis and Theo was not only allowed but crucial to my mental wellbeing. Dave and I cherished and savoured every moment we had that wasn't hospital-based or dominated by the demands of everyday life.

'We could do with a little break,' he'd said. 'Can you get help with the kids next Friday night?'

We arrived at Great Fosters on the Friday afternoon. A spectacular Grade One-listed building set amongst acres of stunning parkland and gardens. I'd never been anywhere like it before. We checked in and then took a walk around the grounds. It was a beautiful warm August day and everything felt perfect.

'Shall we go up to our room?' said Dave as we found ourselves back near the main entrance, having taken in the beauty of outside.

We were staying in the main house and our bedroom was breathtaking. Sixteenth-century tapestries lined the wall, ornate Italian furniture and the highlight – an enormous four-poster bed.

I think it would have been rude of us not to test the mattress, don't you think? Dave pulled a bottle of champagne out of his bag and poured us both a glass.

'I love you so much, baby,' he said, looking into my eyes.

'I love you too,' I replied, almost feeling like I could cry. Had I ever loved this man more than right now, in this very moment? We took the bottle to bed and made love. It felt… different, incredibly intense and I'm not sure I know how to explain why. The emotional intimacy between us was like nothing I'd ever experienced and the need to physically connect overpowering.

Afterwards we lay there feeling closer than ever. Dave topped up our glasses and I luxuriated in the knowledge that we had the whole night and next morning ahead of us in this beautiful, beautiful place. Then Dave got up and walked round to my side of the bed where our bags were and started fumbling around. Yes, he fumbled. He hates that I use that word to describe the magic moment that happened next but it's true! He crouched down, still starkers and *fumbled* around in his case.

'I've got something to ask you,' he said.

Well.

That was it.

I broke down. I sobbed and sobbed and sobbed. Hid my face under the covers and couldn't look at him.

'Hey,' he said as he tried to prise the blankets out of my clenched fists.

'Look at me, darling. I love you so much. I asked your dad too.'

Well.

That finished me off entirely.

I started wailing. He'd asked Dad! My wonderful dad. The man of my life. Until now. The man who'd made it near impossible for any other man to match up.

He leant forward and opened his hand, revealing a small green box.

Cue another ten minutes of hysteria. It took ages before I could look at what was inside. I was overcome. Completely overcome. The ring was beautiful. A princess-cut, platinum ring. It was perfect but, in that moment, it could probably have been a Coke can ring pull or a Haribo jelly ring – my reaction would have been just the same. I spluttered a 'yes' and sobbed some more.

Dave the Carpet. You really did excel yourself that day.

Later that night, after a lot to drink and hours of euphoria we fell drunkenly into bed. Drunk on booze, drunk on love. The next morning we woke to find ourselves covered in brown, sticky stuff. It was everywhere. On us, the sheets, in our hair and all sorts of other nooks and crannies.

What the fuck? We were delirious and confused. Had there been some kind of terrible... accident? What the hell had happened?

We both leapt out of bed, staring at each other's brown bodies. Our heads were pounding, mouths dry – how much did we drink last night? Had there been some kind of mutual bowel explosion?

We pulled back the sheets and shrieked. We'd fallen asleep on a giant opened bag of Maltesers. We'd tossed and turned and they'd rolled around underneath us, crushed and crumbled. We stripped the bed and soaked them in the bath. God knows what the hotel staff thought.

It felt fitting though. Our love was chocolate-covered. I could live with that.

chapter thirty-nine
acceptance

The afternoon before Dave and I got married, Mel and I sat in a coffee bar to grab an hour of calm. It was bedlam back at the house, an absolute tip. We were slap-bang in the middle of the major building work we'd embarked on when Dave moved in and there was dust and debris everywhere. Lola, our eight-week-old Chihuahua, was leaving smelly little presents for us underfoot and the kids were bouncing off the walls, up to their usual tricks as well as being beside themselves with excitement about the big day. In a vague nod to tradition Dave had escaped to stay with Miles for the night and Mel was staying with me as best friend and make-up artist. Miles and Mel were the only two non-family members who would witness our teeny tiny nuptials.

One minute Mel and I were sharing a ridiculously overpriced and tiny piece of Bakewell tart while having a quick run through our last-minute to-do list and the next, much to my mortification, I was blubbering into my almond milk latte and she was scrabbling around in her bag for a Kleenex.

'Darling, what is it?'

I could barely get the words out.

'What *(sob)* if this *(gasp)* isn't it for Dave?' The couple at the next table glanced over and shifted uncomfortably.

'This *(splutter)* is it for me. I'll never be with another man. I love *(sob)* him *(snort)* so much.'

'What do you mean not "it" for Dave? He bloody adores you! What are you talking about?'

It always surprises me that I have to state the obvious to friends and family. Surely they see me as I do? As a woman who's had cancer twice, who's on long-term treatment and who has a much higher than average chance of having the shit hit the fan a third time. Surely they view me as someone who might not be here in five years? Who, most likely, won't be the person they become old and decrepit with? It frustrates me and heartens me at the same time. *Don't you get it?* the frustrated me wants to cry. *Don't you get what it's like to live on borrowed time? Do you have any idea what it's like living inside my head? Do you?*

Deep down I love them for it.

'I never think of you like that, Em,' said Miles once with such conviction that I had no choice but to believe him. 'I can honestly say that I've never once thought that you might not make it.'

Really? REALLY? And it helps, of course it does. But on that day, the eve of my wedding, it was all just too much.

'If I die *(sob)*... if I die he'll find *(splutter)* someone else. He'll have a life with someone else.'

I felt utterly overwhelmed with love for Dave. Of course this was it for me. I'd found him. I'd linked tails with my seahorse and I was done. I felt clear, with every part of me, that my last days would be spent with this man by my side.

But what about him? His romantic future didn't seem as set in stone. On that afternoon, in the state I was in, it didn't seem beyond the realms of possibility that I might one day be in his past. That, one day, after a suitable period of mourning, he might find love again, an even bigger love. What if he found another love and I became just a poignant memory of another life?

'I just want peace,' I gulped as Mel sat listening, her eyes welling up too. 'I would give anything for a break from the constant fear. Especially today... and tomorrow.'

On the eve of my wedding it would have been so nice to have had a temporary respite from thoughts of doom. To instead be thinking only of the many, many years of life that I had no reason to doubt I had before me. Instead I was imagining the attractive, twinkly-eyed divorcee with grown-up kids who might be out there for Dave if I were to die. She'd be free, easy, with no baggage and certainly no Sword of Damocles hovering overhead. That was the very least that he deserved – to marry a woman who he'd got at least a fair to middling chance of growing old with.

Sometimes, as I'm driving over Albert Bridge early on a Tuesday morning on my way to the hospital, I fantasise about simply driving straight past the Royal Marsden and heading somewhere completely different. Where would I go? If I were completely and utterly free to be anyone, go anywhere and do anything without ever giving another thought to cancer – who would I be and how would it feel?

Imagine, Em, just imagine driving away and leaving it all behind. Driving towards peace. Imagine no treatment, no blood tests, no check-ups, no connection at all with a building that is so synonymous with death. Nothing at all in common with Jade Goody, no haunting images of her two boys standing on the front step with their dad in the days before she died. The paparazzi baying, faking sympathy to get the picture that would break a nation's hearts. A tabloid version of Harry and William. She died on Mother's Day, 2009. I remember watching the news on TV and the nation wept and I remember thinking how random life was. That none of us knew what lay ahead. Who's to say it wouldn't be me next year, dead or dying, leaving Jake motherless and alone? One minute a young, feisty woman is exposing her darker side in the *Celebrity Big Brother* house and the next she's almost being canonised by a gripped audience, all waiting with bated breath for her inevitable, tragic and horribly premature passing.

Mother's Day. Those two boys, battered and bewildered. Flown to Australia on the day of the funeral by a father with a perfect understanding of their need for protection, distraction and some kind of hot, sunny normality.

Jake was five back then. Bounding around. I was still just a woman consumed with longing for a baby. That's all I was. Barely a mother, barely a partner, friend, employee, citizen. Self-obsessed and self-absorbed, my body and my womb bullying me, shouting at me to conceive, to reproduce, just one more time.

I'm slowly learning that I can't simply drive past a scary building towards peace. I've probably actually had more tortured moments imagining leaving my kids without a mother while cleaning my teeth than I have had in that building. The fear is in my head. Embedded in every part of me. That doesn't mean it's not real. That doesn't mean that there isn't a high chance that I might face a very dark prognosis at some point over the next few years but I think I've finally realised that I carry the fear, the lack of 'peace' with me wherever I go. And, actually, I've had some extremely peaceFUL moments while sitting hooked up to the IV drip, dunking a bourbon biscuit into my tea feeling perfectly OK. Happy even. My work is to find peace with the fear. To be present with my kids and my husband. To be present with my life, as it is, right now.

There will always be a Royal Marsden in my life. A cancer hospital. It's highly likely that I will always be a patient. Even if the day ever came when I was fortunate enough to be discharged. Even if one day it's decided that I no longer need thrice-weekly treatment, thrice-weekly blood tests and constant, careful monitoring. Then what? What if today, right now, Professor Powles and Mr Sharma from Parkside and Professor Johnston and his team from the Marsden – what if they all lined up smiling and with a high five and a round of applause told me I was free to go? How would I feel? Knowing me, I would feel temporarily euphoric but it wouldn't be long before I found, metaphorically speaking, another 'building of doom'.

Because that's me. That's the way I've been from the very beginning. Maybe cancer isn't my biggest challenge. Maybe my head is my biggest challenge. The prison of my own making, the deaths I die over and over again. On warm sunny spring days when

I'm feeling too low to notice the blossom or on cosy autumnal afternoons when the kids come clattering in with conkers and muddy boots and I shout and scowl because they've invaded my thoughts and crashed into my catastrophising – they're the times when I realise my biggest problem isn't cancer. It's the constant thoughts about cancer. The constant thoughts about the worst happening.

There has to be a freedom within it all otherwise, really, what's the point? What's the point of breakthrough treatments and trials and wonder drugs or the juice, pulp and skin of a thousand organic lemons? What's the point of any of it if my head won't step aside? If I won't get out of my own way?

I've been toying with a new idea and attempting to practise it for quite a while now. *Replacing anxiety with gratitude.* There really is something to it. Just as love and hate can't occupy the same space, neither can anxiety and gratitude. Try it. Try fretting about whatever your 'thing' is. Imagine the worst possible scenario. Go on, colour that image in, turn up the volume, add special effects and put on your 3D glasses. Give that problem all your attention for the next few minutes and then stop. Just say thank you. Quietly. There's no need to try and compete with the main feature presentation. Just say *thank you*.

Something happens, it really does. It might be small but gratitude turns the volume down, it creates space for some kind of happy. For a nugget of peace. I'll take a nugget. Won't you?

chapter forty

yours

It was small, it was intimate, it was the last day of the summer holidays. Monday 5 September, 2016. We were in the iconic and really rather cool Chelsea Registry Office, family only plus Miles and Mel who are as good as. We barely told anyone our plans. I wore a dress from ASOS and earrings from Claire's Accessories because they sparkled like the real thing. Dave went up a notch in a beautiful navy Hugo Boss suit and Ted Baker brogues. Dave's son George looked wonderfully dapper as he always does and as his dad's best man they complemented one another perfectly. By some miracle, Jake agreed to wear a suit and I don't think I'd ever seen him look lovelier. Louis and Theo were prised out of their revolting tracksuit bottoms into their grey school trousers and bribed into wearing shirts which for Louis was utter hell but he did it. Ella discarded her threadbare leggings for the day and embraced her party dress moment, my beautiful, feisty girl.

We'd been living together for nearly a year before our big (little) day and I think we'd both agree that it hadn't been an entirely smooth start. There were huge adjustments to be made on both sides. I think Dave would readily admit that he was mildly traumatised by the shock of moving from a quaint little cottage where he lived in blissful peace to a house that was barely any bigger but housed four unruly kids and had an open-door policy that would on a regular basis turn the living room into the local youth club slash wet play assembly hall.

And the whole step-parent thing. Yikes. Dave arrived with sleeves rolled up, ready to be a strong, loving male figure to my four. Ready to share the load, pick up the slack, instil some much-needed rough and tumble along with a just a tad more discipline. He threw himself into it, gung-ho from the start. He made it all look so easy; he didn't seem to be struggling. Or at least I didn't notice he was struggling and then, a couple of months in, it became clear that he was. Dave was struggling.

We started to row quite a lot. It was a shock. But he carried on, he didn't falter. Up early every morning, hanging the kids upside down by their ankles before leaving for work, sharing the load every single day, sharing the nightly hell of the bedtime routine, sharing the emptying of the dishwasher and the washing machine, accepting that his wife-to-be was no Nigella in the kitchen, that his wife-to-be had never owned an iron and sadly adjusting to the cold, hard fact that his wife-to-be was no longer quite as full of beans in the bedroom. He saw his wife-to-be in her full, knackered, worn-out, granny-knickered glory.

Domestic bliss. Hmm.

We'd gone from our regular bubbles of love at Hotel Belmonte to instant domestic drudgery with, at times, not much in the way of reward.

I loved having him with us, never doubted our decision, but after six years of doing it alone, doing it my way, co-parenting was a shock for me too. I bristled at being challenged on my parenting style. My hackles went up when it was suggested that my way might not be the right way. I resented the occasional implication that maybe my leniency, softness and *oh bugger it, yes have another biscuit and yes, yes watch another hour of telly* survival approach to life with four kids might just be the reason why daily life in the house was So. Flipping. Hard.

But, despite the difficulties, Dave's growing bond with Ella, Louis and Theo was a joy to watch. It happened naturally and him coming into their lives at the age of five meant that they were open to him. They were still in the cuddles, tickles and kisses phase of childhood and their physical closeness inevitably led to genuine stepfather/stepchild love. It hasn't been easy but it's real. The love between Dave and the triplets is definitely real.

With Jake, it's been… trickier. It has taken time. It's still taking time. Jake was eleven when Dave and I met. Twelve when Dave came to live with us and thirteen when we got married. Hardly the easiest of ages.

Dave had high expectations of the two of them becoming mates, having an easy relationship and finding common ground which would help them build a bond unique to them. I also had high hopes of the same and because of that I struggled – still struggle at times – to let them both find their own way with each other. Over time. I've been impatient and frustrated. With both of them.

'Make an effort!' I've shouted at Jake.

'Make an effort!' I've shouted at Dave.

'He's trying really hard!' I've shouted at Jake.

'Can't you try harder?' I've shouted at Dave. 'You're the adult! You have to keep trying!'

'Just leave us to it!' Dave always replies. 'You can't push us together, it'll happen over time.'

And sometimes I leave them to it but more often than not I hover around them both like a human helicopter. Antennae on, ears open, eyes darting between the two 'men' in my life as they battle for space near the toaster or sit in each other's favourite spot on the sofa.

I worry for my boy who hasn't seen his lookalike Papa in years, who isn't into football and banter and wrestling with his inked, strong-armed but highly sensitive stepdad.

Sometimes it's useful to get a fresh perspective. I've seen the same incredible therapist for years. Ever since coming to the end of treatment, first time round. She knows my life and all its issues inside out and upside down. She's been a rock, a constant and (ssh, don't tell her) she's been a friend.

'When you talk about Jake it's as though the two of you got divorced when Dave came along.'

And she's done it again. Nailed it.

Just let them be, Em. Just let them be.

And when I do, it's funny. They actually rub along OK. When I'm not there, hanging around, glaring at Jake for his grunting and scowling at Dave for his strictness, they're OK. They both like steak. Dave cooks a mean steak. Jake makes the best home-made chips in the world. Steak and chips. It's a start.

Our mini wedding day was perfect, as perfect as it could be with a crazy mixed-up family such as ours. Dad and Mum don't seem able to be in the same room as each other so Dad stepped aside and stayed away which was probably for the best. I know how much he loves me and so I didn't push too hard to make him come. Jake walked me down the mini aisle with the biggest smile on his face. 'Our' song, Ella Henderson's 'Yours', played softly in the background, the lyrics so perfectly 'us' that I'd had them framed as a present on our first Valentine's Day together. As we reached Dave, George and the registrar, Jake shook Dave's hand and stepped aside. I cried and Dave cried. We blubbered like babies. Everyone else smiled, huge happy smiles. We were getting married! We were exchanging vows after everything we'd been through and we knew it wouldn't be easy and we didn't know what lay ahead but we knew that this was right. Absolutely, one hundred per cent right.

Mr and Mrs Dave the Carpet. At last. How bloody brilliant.

Afterwards, our mini wedding party stood on the famous town hall steps while a thousand happy photos were taken. Then we hailed three cabs and went for pizza. No frills or fuss, just good food, cheap wine and as much ice cream for the kids as they could eat.

It was perfect. Messy, noisy, chaotic but absolutely perfect.

That night Dave and I went to a local hotel. We sat in bed opening all of the beautiful cards from all of our beautiful friends.

And then I'm sorry but I simply couldn't keep my eyes open.

I fell asleep. Into a deep, deep sleep. Full tummy and full heart.

Bad, bad wife. Poor, poor Dave.

chapter forty-one
the honeymoon blues

Our honeymoon – the honeymoon funded by our wonderful friends, all so happy to see us together – was an absolute disaster for which I take sixty per cent of the blame.

Thirty per cent of the blame lies with both of us for choosing a seriously grim all-inclusive resort in Tenerife and ten per cent lies with Dave for getting really pissed every night and being quite annoying but to be fair, I can't really blame him.

I was in a bad way. Away from home, the familiar routine and the private rituals I have that I like to think keep me sane, I pretty much lost the plot.

Three days before we left it happened again. *No Caller* Flipping *ID*. At work, it was a Friday, no Christmas Jumper on this time but for God's sake, give me a break. I was having a good day! The weekend was going to be busy with preparations and the mammoth task of leaving everything organised for Mum and Miles who were going to share looking after the kids but none of that mattered because we were going on our honeymoon! My mood was particularly buoyant because I'd seen the consultant earlier that week at the hospital and she was really pleased with how I was getting on. She had no concerns. Chemotherapy had finished eighteen months earlier and I was still in remission. The day after seeing her I'd had my bloods taken along with my thrice-weekly dose of Herceptin and so, in principle, I should have been able to switch off from thoughts of cancer for at least a few weeks. Heaven.

And then the missed call happened. And the voicemail.

Dizzy. No, no, no, please not again. The world stopped, again.

It was the hospital asking me to call.

Fuck, fuck, shit, no, no, no, please no...

Shaking, I excused myself from the front desk and found the nearest quiet room to make the call.

'Royal Marsden Medical Day Unit, how can I help?'

'Er, hi it's Emma Campbell – I've had a message to call but I'm not really sure why.'

I could barely breathe while I waited for the nurse to rummage through my notes.

'Oh yes, sorry Emma, there's no problem, we were just ringing to confirm your next appointment in three weeks.'

I put the phone down and felt my knees buckle with relief. I walked back to my desk, breathlessly told my slightly baffled colleagues what had just happened and then went upstairs to make us all a nice cup of tea to celebrate not having been told I was about to die. But by the time the kettle had come to the boil, the feeling of relief had changed into something else. Suddenly I was in more of a state of panic than ever.

Because that's how my mind works. Anxiety, split-second relief and then the triple anxiety hits. This is where the 'madness' kicks in. The understandable insanity but insanity nonetheless.

I then feel the need to tell everyone. To babble deliriously – 'Jeez, you won't believe what just happened!' – and regale them with the HUGENESS of a call from the hospital confirming my routine treatment.

And they politely respond but they don't really get it because there's nothing really to get. Nothing happened. It was as insignificant as a cold call asking me if I'd taken out PPIs in the mid to late nineties.

But I managed, as always, to run with it. To build on something not actually that frightening or threatening and turn it into a tsunami of thoughts. Catastrophic thoughts.

Dipping the last mouthful of a much-needed Twirl bar into my tea was when the mental mayhem really took off and before I knew it I was feverishly trying to come up with the real reason that the hospital had rung. Because I'd decided that there absolutely had to be a reason.

My name has flagged up on the system.

I must have flagged up and it must be my blood results.

They've never rung me to confirm an appointment before. Why would they ring? I have treatment every three weeks and they never, ever ring.

I was spewing out my incoherent thoughts to anyone who would listen, regaling colleagues, tapping out texts to friends with trembling fingers. The sane, sensible, rational responses from my nearest and dearest came back with reassuring speed.

It'll just be an admin thing, Em. Nothing to worry about. Bet you're excited about the honeymoon! Where is it again?

Forget the fucking honeymoon!

Why did they call? Maybe my consultant changed her mind after I left and decided she wasn't so pleased with my progress after all. Maybe she mulled over my notes in her head while she was cooking dinner for her family or bathing her kids. Maybe she couldn't sleep because, actually, something just didn't seem right with me and so she went into work the next day and made a point of going to the Medical Day Unit admin team and asking them to look me up, give me a call and just double check I was definitely going to come in for my next treatment because something might not be right.

That's likely, isn't it? Don't you think? Don't you think something like that must have happened?

You, anyone, everyone could tell me how unlikely that scenario is. But I wouldn't hear you. I wouldn't listen because Cancer, Fear, Terror, whatever you want to call it – the little imp in my mind, the gremlin on my shoulder – can always, *always* talk louder than you. He's right by my ear, inside my head and you, no matter how hard you try, how patient you are, how much you love me, you can't.

You can't make the voice go away.

Only I can do that.

But before that realisation hit, I carried the anxiety and thoughts of dread all the way from the South Terminal at Gatwick Airport to sunny Tenerife. On what should have been the happiest of plane journeys I had an internal, suppressed, panic attack. On the outside I acted all bright and breezy as Dave did his usual thing of flicking through in-flight shopping magazine and perusing the watches and aftershave. On the inside I was longing for a mirror to check how my boobs were looking and feeling. Hoping to steal away when I first had an opportunity. Hoping for relief, however brief. What kind of way was that to start a honeymoon, a new life together?

Two days in, I was reading by the pool, feeling as though every last drop of serotonin had been drained from my brain. I was joyless, foggy. Poor Dave was bewildered and helpless. *You with the sad eyes.* The Cyndi Lauper lyrics regularly played in my head when I looked at the man opposite me. This was the man who had opened his inked arms and let me rest my head. The man who didn't retreat but who had expanded and accepted and wrapped himself around us all. Our grizzly bear at the entrance of the cave. So strong, steady, sore-headed at times but always steady. Always there.

On that holiday, he lost me. I had left the building. My sparkle and smile had diminished along with my libido.

And the kids. My babies. My boy. My horrendous irritability. Screeching at them when they dared to interrupt my thoughts. Leave me alone, I wanted to scream. Leave me alone to obsess and fixate and look and check. Leave me alone so I can stifle my sobs as I imagine leaving you before you are grown. Leave me alone because I'm so scared of leaving you alone that I need to be left alone.

Wow.

And that was how I'd parented the four most precious things in my world. Rarely present or engaged. Time for help. Time for action. Time for acceptance that this couldn't go on.

That's what I realised on my honeymoon with Dave. That I couldn't go on living that way. I needed to get a non-molestation order out on the voices in my head. I needed an indefinite, lifelong, no-contact restraining order on the voices in my poor, frazzled and oh so very afraid head. I needed help. And just like anyone who reaches rock bottom, in any situation, that realisation was a huge, huge relief.

So at some point during our troubled time away, Dave and I agreed that actually our week in Tenerife wasn't our honeymoon after all and that we would rename it. Tenerife was a much-needed change of scene. It was a physical break from our manic lives at home. It gave us crystal clear clarity that all-inclusive, all-you-can-eat buffets displayed in Bain-Maries under hideous fluorescent lights were not for us. It was a holiday. But one thing it most certainly was not was a honeymoon.

We'd have our honeymoon one day. One day when my brain could handle being away from home, away from rituals and obsessions and when different mirrors casting different lights on different parts of my breasts didn't cause quite such high levels of angst.

Something to aim for, don't you think?

chapter forty-two
what's your definition of over?

It's been tough for Dave at times. Really tough. He got so much more than he bargained for when he fell in love with me and I'm not just talking about feral triplets, a tricky teenager and a new life devoid of almost any peace and quiet whatsoever.

For a start, he got a wife who has a big black hole where her brain used to be. I can blame it on lots of things: fourteen cycles of chemo, a medically induced early menopause but most of all (sorry, kiddos) I blame it on my offspring.

My brain is addled.

It's shot to pieces.

It's gone.

'Louis darling, is yours green?'

'No Mummy, it's blue.'

I stand in the bathroom every night and stare at a million toothbrushes. OK, four. A red, a dark blue, a light blue and a green. And every single night I have no idea which colour belongs to which child.

Every night. I know I shouldn't still be putting the toothpaste on their brushes for them. There are *so* many things I shouldn't still be doing for them. The triplets are eight years old for heaven's sake and more than capable. But, while they're faffing around, ignoring everything I say and trying every procrastination trick in the book I just think, to hell with it. It speeds things up and by eight o'clock at night I just need everything to happen really, really quickly. My tank is on empty and the warning light has been flashing for hours.

To me, being a parent to triplets is like playing a lifelong game of Blind Man's Buff. Imagine, if you will, me in the middle of the room (any room) and the kids surrounding me. Theo fixes me with a steely-eyed gaze and reaches into his back pocket to take out a long black scarf. He reaches up and uses it to cover my eyes. Louis assists him by tying it securely so that my world is in complete darkness. Ella walks slowly towards me with that devilish stare of hers (not that I can see it) and reaches up on her tiptoes to put her hands on my shoulders. Slowly, then getting faster, they spin me round and around till I'm so dizzy and disorientated that I almost fall down.

Then the real fun begins. As I'm tripping and stumbling and bumping into things the questions start – firing at me like darts, demanding instant answers and even quicker action.

'Mum, Mum, Mum! Mummy, Mummy, MUMMY!'

And of course Dave is here now and in on the fun. He likens parenting them to standing in front of a faulty tennis ball serving machine. You know the ones. Balls are coming at you from every angle, you're flinching and crouching, ducking and dodging but there's no escape. They just keep coming. And then, at the same time, you're being asked to juggle, or thread a needle, or, or… walk a tightrope. It's just too much. So you collapse, admit defeat and fail at everything.

I don't remember anything any more. If I'm making sandwiches for lunch it's a farce.

'So, kids, can you listen? Kids. Listen! Ella, did you and Theo want ham and cheese and Jake, was it just ham for you and Louis?'

'Yes, Mum. That's right.'

I reach for the bread, start spreading butter on the first slice and –

Dammit. It's gone.

'Theo. THEO! Was it just ham in your sandwich or ham and cheese?'

It's painful. It's embarrassing. It's worrying. But there's nothing I can do. Brain-wise, memory-wise, it's all over for me now. I am that person who freezes the second I'm introduced to someone new. I am that parent who still doesn't know the names of my kids' teachers or which playground mum belongs to which child. I get away with it because I've got the best excuse in the book.

'Oh God, don't worry – you've got triplets! I can't remember anything with just one!'

Phew. That's okay then.

But that's the least of Dave's problems. He's also got a wife who spends an unbearable amount of time thinking she's going to die prematurely. Who worries about everything. Who locks herself in the bathroom so she can examine and study her one 'real' breast while the kids are screaming, fighting and trashing the living room. She's like a secret smoker, a binge eater, drug user or any other kind of addict. She thinks she needs the rituals to somehow keep herself safe.

Insanity is doing the same thing over and over again and expecting a different result.

Dave married a woman who finds it hard to let herself be truly happy because it feels too risky. The more joy, the higher she climbs, the further there is to fall.

There was a defining moment for Dave that took place about six months after we got together. We were in Majorca on our first mini holiday together. I had one more round of chemo to go, seemed to be making very good progress and the next, ongoing phase of treatment was expected to be much less debilitating. It felt as though it wouldn't be long before we could start living a more normal life and really plan our future.

At least I think that's how Dave felt. I was, as always, living day by day, worrying, fretting, fretting, worrying.

We had a lovely time. We sunbathed, swam and read by the pool. We made love in the afternoon and had candlelit meals at night. We were still learning about each other, confident that what we had was real but probably also deciding whether the niggles could be lived with, whether what we had was really going to last. There ain't nothing like a holiday to help you decide if you're destined to be more than once-a-week companions.

We were a couple of days in and just starting to really relax. I had some colour in my washed-out cheeks and even though having chemo meant I had to be careful of having too much sun, I could still feel the warmth and sunshine doing my worn-out body so much good.

I was showered, I'd done my best to make my straggly, thinning hair look decent and was sitting on the balcony with a glass of wine while Dave finished getting ready.

Then I happened to pick up my phone and open Facebook. Scrolling down, my right thumb hovered over a video of a lady with no hair. Scroll on, Em. Just scroll on. But of course I couldn't. I watched the thirty-second film. She was a mum and had secondary breast cancer. It was one of those 'hit "like" to save this poor lady' type of things. I hate them. How can anyone's life be reduced to a thousand, a million likes?

I shuddered and put the phone face down back on the table.

Shake it off, Em. Shake it off. It's not you, not your story.

Dave appeared from behind me, bending down to kiss the back of my neck.

'Ready, angel?'

'Yeah,' I said, standing up. 'Just seen something really depressing on Facebook. A cancer video – really wish I hadn't looked.'

Dave looked at me and gave a really heavy sigh. 'Why do you do it to yourself, darling? Why do you watch things like that?'

I shrugged and stood up.

'Obligatory hotel balcony selfie before we go?'

We wrapped our arms round each other and smiled our best smiles. The happy couple on holiday. The happy, soon-to-be healthy couple on holiday. Could that be true? He believed it so why couldn't I?

Later on, sitting in a bar having a pre-dinner drink, we were both unusually quiet.

'You OK?' I finally asked. He had that rabbit in the headlights look I'd come to know meant there was something on his mind.

'It's never going to be over, is it?'

'What do you mean?'

'Cancer. You and cancer.'

I didn't say anything.

'I thought that chemo would finish and that would be it. We could move on and leave it behind. Seeing the way you reacted to that Facebook video brought it home to me just how much it's a part of you, of us.'

I didn't know what to say and when I finally did speak my reply was damaging. More damaging than I realised.

'I've had cancer twice. How on earth can it ever be over?'

Dave looked shattered.

'But you've done so well. Everyone is so pleased with your progress. You've beaten it twice. Surely we can try to move on, put it in the past?'

I spent a great deal of the first year of our relationship feeling wretchedly guilty that I'd somehow tricked Dave, lied to him and lured him into my lair without laying out the bare facts. He seemed so hopeful, so optimistic but, to me, so in denial.

I spoke to close friends about it. To my therapist.

'Should I tell him?' I'd say. 'Should I gently break the news to him that "this" might not be "it"? That I might get ill again and die? I don't think he realises; how can he not realise?'

And each time the answer would be the same.

'Em. Darling. He's a grown man. He's been with you every step of the way. He knows. You haven't lied to him, or tricked him. He knows what could happen and he made a choice.'

'Really?' I'd reply. 'Do you really think so?'

'Yes,' they'd all say. 'And do you know what, Em? You might stay healthy. This might just be the end of your cancer story.'

Well. Now there was a thought I hadn't ever let myself think.

chapter forty-three
now

December 2017

As your kids get older and your friends' kids get older too you find that being around tiny babies is a rare thing. Gone are the days of comparing pregnancy bump sizes, baby wipes spilling out of your handbag and random fluff-covered dummies popping up where you least expect them. Sticky spillages on your shoulder are a distant memory as are endless extremely dull discussions about formula or weaning techniques. In lots of ways you're glad to see the back of it all and move the hell on. Having spent four years utterly consumed with longing for another baby my broodiness disappeared the second the triplets were born. I was clearly done. Done, I tell you. Done, du-done, done, done.

The other day I got to cuddle a five-week-old baby girl called Blossom. The new baby daughter of a friend of mine. It was one of the very few times I'd properly held a tiny baby since Ella, Louis and Theo were born. I could have sobbed. That would have been a dramatic, unnecessary and rather embarrassing reaction but it knocked me for six. Holding this gorgeous little bundle, hearing her funny little noises, breathing in her milky smell, her tiny fingers curled around mine and all I could think was – *I don't remember holding my three like this*. I don't remember. All I remember was stress and pushing on through to the next feed, the next nappy change, the next pocket of sleep. I DON'T REMEMBER THE GOOD BITS and that is devastating.

Blossom gazed up and fixed her eyes on mine. I fed her a bottle of milk and winded her afterwards, muslin over my shoulder like an old pro. Why can't I remember feeding my Ella? Why can't I remember just sitting with Theo curled up like a hibernating hedgehog on my chest? Why can't I remember the precious moments that made all the other stuff bearable?

'Daytime telly. That's all I'm doing. Watching daytime telly, eating biscuits and hanging out with Blossom,' said Janna, her lovely mum, and my heart cracked a little bit more.

Hanging out with Blossom.

Just hanging out. Just hanging… Heaven.

So how is life now?

It's certainly different.

I often drive past the old flat. Our home at the top of a million stairs. I'll find myself sitting in traffic, heading towards Clapham Common and just a few feet away from our old life.

If I look to my right straight up at the kitchen window that overlooks the street I can picture Marc leaning out, smoking a cigarette. I can almost see him smile and wave at me, just like he must have done a thousand times during the seven years we were together.

We fell in love in that flat, made Jake there, fought and battled there. There are a thousand happy memories and just as many grim ones. I don't know what to make of it any more. Of us. Of the man who shared my life for seven years. I regularly dream that we've met again and all is well. All is calm with no more fights. No more fear. We're friends. I dreamt recently that Marc met Dave and shook him by the hand, happy that a good, good man had appeared in the lives of his four beautiful kids. I liked that dream.

That flat turned from my solitary haven into our shared love nest and then slowly but surely into a prison of our own making.

Sometimes, if Jake's in the car with me, we'll both look up and touch on a memory.

'Mum, do you remember when…?'

And, depending on the moment he recalls, I'll either smile or shudder. There's a real nostalgia. I loved that flat and for a time, our life there.

If Ella, Louis and Theo are with us in the car we'll all find ourselves looking up while waiting for the traffic lights to change from red to green.

'Look darlings, that's where we all used to live.'

'I don't remember, Mummy, why don't I remember?'

And I'm relieved that they don't remember. And sad too. Because there were good times there. And a lot of love. And so many dreams. Intense, longed for, intricately detailed dreams.

I got what I wanted, didn't I? I got my baby. Babies. I got the noise and the chaos and the mess and the family life I spent years dreaming about.

Cancer came and it made everything worse but better too.

Cancer lingers on. Not active as I write – thank you, thank you, thank you – but always there, wreaking havoc in my mind if not currently in my body.

But I am trying. Really, I am.

I'm doing my best to live a full, authentic, big, strong life. To be less afraid, more light-hearted, to laugh more and believe that it's safe to let myself be truly happy. To recognise that finding more moments of happiness does not equal disaster striking. That belly laughs won't set off a chain of catastrophic events. That I'm safe – as safe as any of us can be.

I'm working on being the mother that my miracle babies deserve. I want Ella, Louis and Theo to have the me that Jake used to have. For Jake to have the me that he once had, before everything happened.

I want my darling Dave to feel that he made the right choice. I remember that day when he walked me to the car and saw three baby seats in a row, that day when he stood at a crossroads. Which path should he choose? He chose the difficult one. The one full of trickiness and challenges and risks and long periods of time where there seems to be little reward. But I hope, with all of my heart, that he feels that he chose the right path for him. The path that, despite everything, is paved, etched, cemented with love. Real, solid, tested, evolving love.

And I'm a stepmother too. A stepmum! To lovely George, Dave's grown-up boy. How funny and unexpectedly lovely. He's adored by the little ones and edged around by Jake. Jake edges around everyone these days. I'm not sure if that's him being a teenager or because he feels happier, safer when he keeps his distance. I hope it's the former. I miss my golden-haired, smiley nature boy. I've struggled for so long with the feeling that I let him down – turned his life upside down in a way that I thought couldn't be rectified. But then we had a conversation that healed me more deeply than hours of therapy and angst has ever done.

Dave was away filming a makeover. The triplets were in bed. It had been another tough patch at home, every day a hard slog with not much in the way of light relief. I'd been crying a lot. Weeping. Hospital anxiety, the triplets' reign of terror and the honeymoon period feeling like a distant memory for a worn-out Dave and me.

Jake sat by my side, just like the old days – a family-sized bar of chocolate half eaten on the table, *Made in Chelsea* on catch-up – and then unexpectedly we found ourselves pressing pause on the remote and talking more intimately than we had in years.

Jake was unusually emotional. He'd spent the day with Dad – his beloved, adored grandad – and a rare glimpse of him seeming frail, looking his years, had knocked Jake. The tears flowed. I hadn't seen Jake properly cry for longer than I could remember.

'Today made me realise that Grandad won't be around forever,' he said, hiding his contorted face with his arm and burying his head in his knees, huddled on the sofa.

I moved closer to him and held him tight, part of me grateful for his tears as they allowed me to show him physical warmth and affection, something so rarely permitted these days.

After a few moments of talk and tears I touched on the one subject that I'd always avoided. It suddenly felt crucial that I knew how much anxiety my eldest boy might be carrying, if any, about me.

'Do you ever worry about my health, darling?'

'Not really,' he replied, rubbing his face. 'Maybe about once a week.'

I had no sense of whether Jake thinking about me and cancer once a week was good or bad. Once a week compared to my own constant negative internal chatter is bloody brilliant – I would give anything to have thoughts of cancer on a weekly rather than hourly basis. But once a week compared to his school friends, other teenage boys with not much on their minds other than girls and Snapchat, is once a week too much. It's too much heaviness for a young boy who used to have the lightest of hearts.

We talked some more, the tears dried and our chat moved onto the subject of home life, the craziness, noise, stress and mayhem.

'I'd hate to be an only child though, Mum.'

That sentence stopped me in my tracks.

'You'd hate to be an only child?'

'I'd hate it! It would be awful!'

'But, but, but' – the spluttering started – 'I thought you resented the little ones, blamed them for everything changing, for me and Papa, for the chaos –'

'Of course not, Mum. Don't be silly! I love them! I hate it when they're not here. The house is really quiet and boring and I know they're really annoying but they're pretty great really, aren't they?'

I wiped my nose on my dressing-grown sleeve, a habit picked up from Louis, and snivelled a response.

'Yes, they are. And *(uh-oh, off again)* it's *(sob)*... not *(splutter)*... their *(sniff)* fault.'

I cried like a baby. Like a big blubbering baby. Poor Jake. Poor Ella, Louis and Theo. Poor Dave. Poor Marc even. What a flipping mess it's all been.

'It's OK Mum. Don't cry. It's OK.' He even leant towards me and gently put a hand on my knee. Jake who hasn't let me hug him properly for about two years.

'I'm sorry, Jakey. I'm sorry it's all been so hard. Still is so hard. I love all of you so much.'

'I know you do, Mum. We know you do. And it's okay. You don't need to feel bad. We're all okay.'

And right now I think we really are all okay. And we keep trying, because that's all any of us can do, don't you think?

And there is so, so, so much good to be found. In the madness. The darkness. My challenge, in this lifetime, is to gently put the fear to one side and look up. Look around. I got my babies! Fuck cancer. They came! They're here and they are a marvel.

How lucky am I?

I hope you feel it from me, my beautiful four. I hope that every single day you can feel my love and see past the furrowed brow, the irritability and intolerance. Because despite your tricky ways, the challenges you bring, the energy you deplete, my sadness or anger is never because of you. Not really. Not deep down below the superficial mess and clutter and tantrums. My times spent hiding away are never because of you. OK? It's my stuff. And I'm trying, every day, to be better than before so that I can feel proud of the mum I am and that you can feel proud of me.

Oh, and also because I really want you to look after me when I'm old.

Because I plan to get really, really old.

Do you hear me, kids?

Mummy isn't going anywhere.

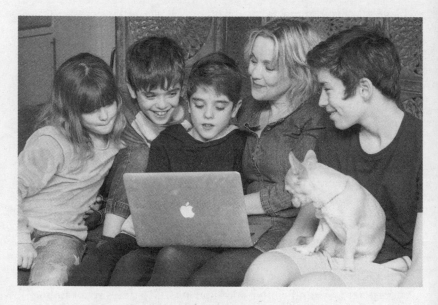

April 2018. Oh, how they've grown.

acknowledgements

Where do I begin in attempting to thank all of those who have shown such love and care over the last eight years? I'm very aware that I haven't come close to sharing every act of kindness in this book and that only a fraction of what happened has made the final edit. But there are so many amazing people who are a part of this story. So many hands reached out to hold mine, to soothe a crying baby, to bake a hearty lasagne for the freezer and to push that bloody giant buggy wherever it needed pushing.

To Katy and my rota angels: Amber, Liz, Becca, Katherine, Kerry, Jo, Dawn, Celia, Eilish and Julie. To Karen and Maria, for going above and beyond in ensuring I found a way to sleep during the chemo months.

Thank you Camilla and Robert for bringing Connie into our lives. Thank you Connie, Em, Lucia, Leny and Daniela for all the love and help.

Thank you to Sheila, the maternity nurse who saved the day.

Thank you to Jessie, Esther, Ali, Eileen, Deardra, Hannah and to my Pacellini family – Steph, Sophie and Lara. Thank you to the Facebook Multiple Mums who rallied round in the most generous way. To Lou and Jim for your incredible generosity and to all the lovely neighbours who made a bald lady with four kids so welcome on the close.

Thank you darling Lucy for 'marrying' Dave and me for the second time in such a perfect way – I'm so happy that we share our beautiful 'quads'.

Thank you to Mel, Miles, Geoff and Eileen, my Yorkshire family. Mel, what can I say and where to begin? Don't know where I'd be without you. Miles, the countless hours you've spent with Ella, Louis and Theo are so appreciated, as is your unconditional love and support – thank you my 'face the east' friend. Love you both.

And huge, grateful, giddy thanks to my fantastic agent Jon Elek at United Agents. And to his team (past and present), Millie Hoskins, Kat Aitken and Rosa Schirenberg. Your support and belief in me has made writing this book the most incredible experience and I feel so, so lucky to be able to call myself a client.

Thank you to Ros Powell for the early reads and spot-on editing and huge thanks to Jo, Paula and the fantastic Mirror Books team. Working with you has been a dream, can we do it again please?

To all of my colleagues at United Agents, from reception on the ground floor to those up on the fourth. Special thanks to Thea for instigating so much help and to my long-suffering but wonderful reception colleagues – Jan, Janna, Sally, Terry and Sara – for putting up with me on those foggy-brained, worn-out, good-for-nothing days. I couldn't be prouder to be part of such an incredible company. Thank you for the cake bakes, the time off and for always welcoming me back with open arms.

To Peter Andre, Ben Hillman, ITV and the '60 Minute Makeover' team! You transformed our house and you led me to Dave the Carpet. What an unexpected bonus that was!

To all of my amazing Wimbledon Rock Choir Friends: Jim, Helen, Linda, Christine, Zoe, Michelle, Sharon, Tony and the gang. You gave me a new lease of life when I needed it most and kindness and care when I needed it even more.

Thank you to all of the incredible staff and volunteers at Home-Start Wandsworth. In particular, Kelly, Amelia, Lisa, Wendy and Judy.

And Sue. My lovely friend Sue. I miss you.

To my wonderful therapist Bernadette Knight, you've supported me so much, thank you.

Special thanks, love and appreciation to Professor Trevor Powles, Mr Anup Sharma and all of the amazing staff at the Cancer Centre London and Parkside Hospital. And to Professor Stephen Johnston, his team and all of the incredible nurses in the Medical Day Unit at the Royal Marsden in Fulham. I know I'm in the best hands, always have been.

And lastly, but absolutely not least, thank you to Dad, Mum, Fiona and Ro. We're a bonkers family but I wouldn't change a thing and I honestly don't know where I'd be without you all. Sorry for giving you all so many sleepless nights. I love you all very, very much.

Please, please forgive me if I haven't mentioned everybody who should be mentioned or you've remembered events differently from the way I've described them here. Chemo brain is a real thing, honest ;) Love you all. Em xx

www.meandmyfour.com
Instagram: @emplus54

Also by Mirror Books

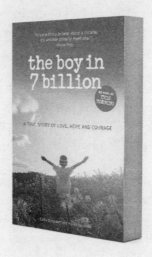

The Boy in 7 Billion
Callie Blackwell and Karen Hockney

If you had a chance to save your dying son... wouldn't you take it?

Deryn Blackwell is a walking, talking miracle. At the age of 10, he was diagnosed with Leukaemia. Then 18 months later he developed another rare form of cancer called Langerhan's cell syndrome. Only five other people in the world have it. He is the youngest of them all and the only person in the world known to be fighting it alongside another cancer, making him one in seven billion. Told there was no hope of survival, after four years of intensive treatment, exhausted by the fight and with just days to live, Deryn planned his own funeral.

But on the point of death – his condition suddenly and dramatically changed. His medical team had deemed this an impossibility, his recovery was nothing short of a miracle. Inexplicable. However, Deryn's desperate mother, Callie, was hiding a secret...

Callie has finally found the strength and courage to reveal the truth about Deryn's battle. The result is a book that everyone should read. It truly is a matter of life and death.

Also by Mirror Books

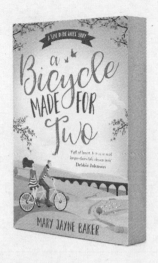

A Bicycle Made for Two
A Love In The Dales story...
by Mary Jayne Baker

In a lost corner of the Yorkshire Dales, Lana Donati runs a medieval theme tourist trap restaurant with her brother. As a distraction to help them get over losing the father they loved dearly, and as a tribute to his passion for the beautiful area they live in, Lana hatches a plan to boost business for everyone by having the Grand Départ route pass through their village.

This means getting the small community to work together to make it happen – including arrogant celebrity Harper Brady and Lana's (attractive) arch-nemesis – the former pro-cyclist turned bike shop owner Stewart McLean, whose offbeat ideas might just cost them everything.

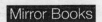